ATKINS DIET COOKBOOK

The Easy Steps to Follow Guide to Understand Atkins Meal Plan

(Beginners Guide on Shedding Weight and Living Healthy)

Robert Decker

Published by Alex Howard

© **Robert Decker**

Atkins Diet Cookbook: The Easy Steps to Follow Guide to Understand Atkins Meal Plan (Beginners Guide on Shedding Weight and Living Healthy)

ISBN 978-1-990169-67-0

Legal & Disclaimer

The information contained in this book is not designed to replace or take the place of any form of medicine or professional medical advice. The information in this book has been provided for educational and entertainment purposes only.

Table of contents

Part 1...1

Introduction 2

Chapter 1 - the atkins diet 3

Chapter 2 - how does it work?..5

Chapter 3 - what are the benefits?..7

Chapter 4 - guidelines in following the atkins diet.........10

Chapter 5 - atkins meal guide 14

Chapter 6 - the new atkins diet meal plan 20

Chapter 7 - atkins diet for life 25

Chapter 8: desserts recipes...29

Dark Mocha Pudding...29

Decadent Chocolate Cake...30

Decadent Chocolate Ice Cream 32

Double Chocolate Cookies 33

Earl Grey Tea and Chocolate Pots de Crème......................34

Endulge Chocolate Cups 36

Endulgent Chocolate-Covered Strawberries 36

Extra-Creamy Strawberry Shake..37

Firecracker Popsicles...38

Fresh Berry Tarts with Cream 39

Frozen Chocolate Fudge Tart...40

Frozen Peanut Butter Chocolate Cheesecake Bombs.......41

Frozen Peppermint Pie 43

Ginger Flan..44

Ginger Ice Cream with Caramelized Pears 45

Holiday Cookies...46

Indulgent Espresso Chocolate Cake 47

Irish Coffee 49

Lemon Mousse 49

Low Carb Pumpkin Pecan Cheesecake 51

Low-Carb Chocolate Blueberry Cheesecake Tartlets 52

Mascarpone Parfait 54

Mexican Hot Chocolate Souffle 55

Mixed Berry Shortcakes 56

Mocha Granita 57

Mocha-Hazelnut Ice Cream 58

Molten Chocolate Cake 60

Old Fashioned Bread Pudding 61

Panna Cotta 62

Passover Angel Food Cake with Rhubarb-Strawberry Sauce 63

Peach-Buttermilk Sherbert 64

Peanut Butter and Jelly Thumbprints 65

Pear Tart 67

Peppermint-Chocolate Truffles 68

Pineapple-Coconut Granita 69

Pineapple-Mango Layer Cake 71

Pinwheel Cookies 72

Pistachio Butter Cookies 74

Pumpkin Cheesecake 75

Pumpkin Mousse 76

Pumpkin Pie Topped with Meringue and Toasted Nuts 77

Pumpkin Pie with Pecan Crust 79

Pumpkin Pots 81

Pumpkin-Spice Brownies...82

Raspberry Parfait..84

Root Beer Float...85

Snickerdoodle Cupcakes..86

Spiced Coconut Bark..88

Spiced Snack Cake 89

Star Spangled Berry Trifle..90

Strawberries and Cream Cupcakes 93

Strawberries with French Cream....................................94

Strawberry Granita 95

Strawberry Shortcake Trifle...96

Strawberry-Rhubarb Pie 98

Sweet Potato-Pumpkin Purée..99

Tiramisu Cupcakes..100

Tropical Raspberry Smoothie.......................................102

Truly Coconut Cake...103

Vanilla Mousse with Rhubarb Sauce 104

Vanilla-Almond Butter Cookies....................................105

Vanilla-Bean Biscotti...107

Vanilla-Coconut Ice Cream 108

Vegan Coconut-Vanilla Shake 109

Walnut Blondies 109

Walnut Brownies 111

Part 2...113

Introduction 114

Chapter 1: background of the atkins diet......................116

Chapter 2: the atkins diet explained............................120

Chapter 3: advantages and disadvantages of atkins diet......123

Chapter 4: the different phases of the atkins diet...................127

Chapter 5: benefits of the atkins diet 132

Chapter 6: atkins diet food lists 134

Chapter 7: steps to starting atkins diet 137

Chapter 8: approved and unapproved atkins diet foods......140

Atkins recipes 148

Low Carb Asian Whole Fried Snapper..............................148

Low Carb Cilantro Lime Fish..149

Zero Carb Grilled Parmesan Encrusted Tilapia...................150

Zero Carb Lobster Dip 151

Zero Carb Smoked Spanish Mackerel or Mullet...................152

Low Carb Ceviche..153

Low Carb Fried Clams...154

Low Carb Grouper Fingers...155

Low Carb Lobster Salad 156

Zero Carb Parmesan Encrusted Tilapia 157

Zero Carb Balsamic Salmon..158

Zero Carb Blackened Fish 159

Low Carb Blackened Scallops 160

Low Carb Cajun Shrimp...161

Low Carb Classic Tuna Salad...162

Zero Carb Crab Cakes..163

Zero Carb Dijon Salmon Bake 164

Zero Carb Drawn Butter...165

Low Carb Fried Calamari..166

Zero Carb Fried Fish...167

Low Carb Fried Oysters 168

Zero Carb Fried Shrimp 169

Zero Carb Garlicky Blue Crabs 170

Low Carb Grilled Parmesan Oysters 171

Low Carb Grilled Salmon 172

Zero Carb Shrimp Scampi 173

Zero Carb Lobster On The Grill 173

Low Carb Oyster Stew 174

Low Carb Oysters On The Half Shell 174

Low Carb Oysters Rockefeller 175

Zero Carb Salmon Cakes 176

Low Carb Seared Scallops 176

Low Carb Italian Shrimp Alfredo 177

Zero Carb Shrimp Cocktail 178

Low Carb Smoked Fish Dip 178

Low Carb Snow Crab Legs 179

Low Carb Steamed Clams 180

Zero Carb Steamed Lobster 181

Low Carb Tartar Sauce 181

Zero Carb Tuna Steaks 182

Low Carb Tuna Tartar 182

Low Carb Land and Sea Salad 183

Low Carb Australian Style Snapper 184

Low Carb French Baked Scallops 185

Low Carb African Fried Fish Balls 185

Conclusion 187

Part 1

Introduction

Within this book you will find Everything you need to know about the Atkins Diet. Including recipes, meal strategies and the basics of thought to help you on your journey to achieving your ideal weight. Moreover, in this book you will get the insight on how to stick with the diet after you do achieve your ideal weight, unlike most every other diet book out there. The real secret is how to keep the weight off and keep it off! All the while in this dieting journey in which you are about to embark upon, enjoying the foods that YOU REALLY LIKE TO EAT!

This book contains proven steps and strategies on how the Atkins diet can change your life. The main focus of this book is on making this diet a part of your lifestyle. Here are the different meal plans and strategies to live a full life following this diet. Read on and find out how to live healthier and happier with Atkins diet.

If you are like so many others out there, that has tried every diet that is popular and do not see the results, this book is for You!

If you struggle to lose weight, this book is for You!

If you get bored with restrictive diets, this book is for You!

If you have struggled with your weight and cannot seem to keep the weight off, this book is for You!

There are many diets out there, but none of them is like the Atkins Diet!

Chapter 1 - the atkins diet

Officially named as Atkins Nutritional Approach, the Atkins diet that was first introduced by Robert Atkins in 1958. A weight reduction technique follows a low carbohydrate diet. Its basic principle is limiting the intake of carbohydrates. The body's main sources of energy are carbohydrates and fat. Burning carbohydrates as energy is faster than burning fats. The more glucose in the blood, the more energy is available to the cells. By reducing the intake of carbohydrates, the body is forced to turn to burning the stored fats for energy. Hence, the body will lose weight as more stored fats are utilized or burned off. According to Dr. Atkins, more calories are needed to burn fats, so the body's calorie burn rate is doubled. Hence, the body benefits a lot with a low carbohydrate diet.

The Atkins diet has been introduced as a weight loss program that only focuses on the effects of carbohydrates in the body. The follower of this diet only has to cut back on the carbohydrate intake, and not on other food types. Proteins and fats have been encouraged. Fats have long been held as a bad for the health. In Atkins diet, fats are essentially part of the daily meal. This is in complete contrast to most diets that say no to fats in the diet. In Atkins, eat that you want, even the labeled "rich" foods like creams and fats. This program lets you enjoy the food, only watch the carbohydrates. Hence, eat while you lose weight. There is no need for starving yourself.

The Atkins diet is controversial because it only puts focus on the amount of carbohydrate intake. Proteins, fibers and fats are not strictly controlled nor prohibited. These are even encouraged. Proteins and fats take longer time to digest therefore hunger is delayed. Fibers are not digestible at all, but add to the amount or bulk in the stomach. This bulk delays the hunger sensation. The net carbohydrate content of food is calculated in the Atkins diet. It is simply subtracting the amount of fiber and sugar alcohols from the total carbohydrate count of a food item.

Chapter 2 - how does it work?

The Atkins diet is training the body to become a fat-burner and not to heavily rely on carbohydrates for fuel. The carbohydrate intake is drastically reduced. Stay away from carbohydrate-rich foods like refined sugar, white flour, and white rice. Eat more of proteins and fats. The diet allows eating most foods that are traditionally labeled as rich like eggs, cheese, and meat.

You are actually encouraged to eat more of these over carbohydrates. This is to achieve two things. One, it is to reduce the carbohydrate dependency of the body. Two, it can help decrease the appetite. Proteins and fats are more difficult to digest than carbohydrates. It takes a longer time for the digestive system to breakdown these food groups. Hence, hunger sensation is delayed. In addition, the rich fiber content of the foods in Atkins diet reduces the cravings. Fiber is not digestible, but adds to the feelings of stomach heaviness and fullness after a meal. It generally stays longer in the digestive system; hence, one feels full longer.

High carbohydrate meals results to increased blood sugar levels. The body responds by secreting more insulin. This enzyme regulates the blood sugar by storing some of it into the liver. Whatever sugar the liver cannot store is quickly converted into fat. The more carbohydrates you consume, the more insulin is released. As a result, more of the blood glucose becomes converted into fat. There is a cycle of more eating, more insulin, more fat stored, more cravings. In Atkins diet, the carbohydrate intake is drastically reduced. The body is reprogrammed to turn from a carbohydrate consumer to a fat burner. The body is placed in a ketotic state. It is stimulated to burn fats to generate energy. This process of fat burning is called lipolysis. It is induced when the body has low insulin levels because of low glucose in the blood. Fat burning produces ketones. In the presence of ketones, the body feels less hungry.

Proteins, along with fats, are encouraged in the Atkins diet plan. It is a very important macronutrient in the body. It is needed in every aspect of bodily function. Among these functions is the maintenance of normal metabolism. Enzymes and hormone production need the presence of proteins. Growth and repair of tissues are also aided by proteins. In the regulation of hunger, proteins help you feel more satisfied with a meal. It is digested more slowly, delaying hunger. Main protein sources are all forms of animal meats like beef, pork, fish, and poultry. It is also present in animal by-products like milk, cheese, and eggs. Vegetables can also provide proteins. These include legumes, seeds, and nuts. Proteins have less influence over insulin. It exerts more control over glucagon. This hormone promotes the release of energy by burning stored fat. Proteins also promote increased metabolic rate. In Atkins diet, the amount of protein in each meal should be at least 6 oz.

Fat is not a bad in the system. While there are bad fats, there are also good ones. Natural fats like saturated fats are actually necessary for good health. It provides protection to vital organs by acting as a shock absorber and insulator. Vitamins, particularly fat-soluble cannot be absorbed in the absence of fats. The body utilizes fats as back up energy source. Fats also add flavor to food. It increases the feeling of satiety. With these benefits, fat is not necessary to be eliminated from the food intake, like most diet plans claim.

Chapter 3 - what are the benefits?

The Atkins diet is primarily a weight loss regimen. The effect on the body does not stop there. As the body loses weight through fat burning, a series of chemical reaction is triggered. The by-products of these reactions cause another series of reactions. Simply put, the biochemical process that the Atkins diet triggers a cascade of reactions that ultimately benefit the body. Severely restricting the carbohydrate intake for the first 2 weeks forces the body to enter the ketogenic phase. The body responds by releasing growth hormones and epinephrine. Metabolism increases in the presence of these hormones. The fat-burning cycle stimulated by the Atkins diet helps reduce the risk for cardiovascular diseases.

Weight loss is the main benefit from following the Atkins diet. The body burns the fat when there is very little carbohydrate from food intake. Weight maintenance is more achievable with the Atkins diet. You are actually looking for just the right amount of carbohydrates that your body needs for every single day. The Atkins diet program starts from a minimal carbohydrate intake. Then, gradually increasing to a level wherein it neither cause weight gain nor weight loss. With the whole program, dieters are encouraged to eat nutritious food that contains the more important nutrients and vitamins.

Low-density lipoprotein (LDL) decreases, and the good cholesterol HDL (high-density lipoprotein) increases with the Atkins diet. There is significant increase in the body's triglyceride levels, which is linked to a decreased risk in developing cardiovascular diseases. Consequently, reduction of cholesterol in the body also decreases the blood pressure.

Insulin activity is better regulated. When the body is subjected to constantly high blood glucose, more insulin is released. Over time, the body develops a resistance to insulin, making it ineffective at lowering blood glucose. Insulin resistance improves when carbohydrate intake is restricted. A study shows that insulin resistance is better improved in Atkins diet than when following low fat and calorie restricted diets. With better insulin regulation and function, the body has a lower risk of developing diabetes.

The Atkins diet is cutting back only on carbohydrates. There is still a wide selection of foods that are allowed and still may cause you to lose weight. Food can even be made more interesting through spices and herbs. There is also less possibility of overeating.

The body is trained to be less reliant on carbohydrates for fuel. Carbohydrate as fuel subjects the body to alternate burst of energy and energy drain. The body quickly metabolizes the carbohydrate and converts it to glucose. If there is no immediate need, it is also quickly stored. Proteins and fats on the other hand, are more stable energy sources. They are digested slowly. The energy is also released slowly. The body has a steady supply of energy, given at a stable pace. Trained in this manner, the body operates in a relatively steady manner. This way, the cravings for quick energy like sugary foods are lessened. Protein and fats in the meals are more filling and satisfying. These types of foods tend to keep the blood sugar at a constant level. The spikes in the blood sugar throughout the day are avoided. Hence, you tend to have more energy. The energy drain, especially in the afternoons will gradually fade away. Emotional and compulsive eating are also reduced. There is also better brain function because of the steady and stable supply of energy to the brain.

The Atkins diet is not free from negative effects on the body. The drastic drop in the carbohydrate intake during the induction phase will cause a few health complaints. Headache and dizziness are typical in the induction phase as the body is not used to the low blood sugar levels. Weakness and easy fatigability can also result from the low carbohydrate intake. Most carbohydrate rich foods are also high in fiber. Restricting these mean eating less fiber. Constipation is likely to result from very little fiber intake. The body gets too little nutrients from the restricted diet. The dieter is advised to take nutritional supplements to address the body's needs.

The ketotic stage is so named because of the release of ketones as a by-product of fat burning. Ketones in the body can lead to headaches and mental fatigue. There is also feeling of nausea. The breath has this fruity acetone quality, or termed ketone breath.

Some experts say that high protein diet can increase the risk of developing kidney problems like stones. This diet is not recommended for people with a prevailing kidney problem. It can worsen and lead to kidney failure. Gout can also worsen with high protein meals.

The severe cutting back on carbohydrate intake causes a big drop in the blood sugar in the early stages. Consult your doctor before starting this diet most especially so if you have diabetes or insulin issues.

*This diet is only not recommended for pregnant and breastfeeding women. Nutrient intake is at a minimum, which can affect the baby. *

Chapter 4 - guidelines in following the atkins diet

For the first two weeks, you will be eating only about 20 grams of net carbohydrates. As such, weight-loss biochemical activity is jumpstarted. There is no need to count the calorie intake. Only put focus on the net carbohydrates. This part of the Atkins diet plan is the induction phase. The body is forced to enter the ketogenic phase. The carbohydrate intake is drastically reduced to force the body to turn to burning fat. The blood glucose levels need to be reduced to less than 64.5 mg/dL (3.58 mmol/L). With this amount, the body is stimulated to release epinephrine, growth hormones, and glucagon to maintain metabolism. Epinephrine and growth hormones enter the adipose cells and stimulate the breakdown of triacylglycerol. A cascade of reactions ensues, resulting to the release of ketones and dissolution of the fat cell.

The induction phase diet consists of mainly vegetables. The original list by Dr. Atkins consists of only 54 allowed food. Most of them are salad greens and vegetables like broccoli, pumpkin, asparagus, and turnips. Legumes are excluded because they contain a lot of starch. About 2 to 3 cups loosely heaped with the salads are allowed. You can also include 4 to 6 ounces of all types of meats, eggs, fish, shellfish, fowl, and poultry. Cheeses are also allowed but only up to 4 ounces per day. Caffeine is permitted only if it does cause low blood sugar levels or create cravings for sweets. It should be taken in moderation. Because of the severe restriction on carbohydrates and limited list of fruits and vegetables, you should start taking multivitamin supplements. Those that contain iron are avoided.

Normally, in the induction phase, food is composed of 20 grams of natural sugars from vegetables, 150 grams of protein and at least 100 grams of fats. Proteins include all fish and seafood. These are essentially carbohydrate free. Oysters and mussels should be eaten in moderation because they contain carbohydrates. At this phase, significant weight loss is commonly observed. You may lose about 5 to 10 pounds per week due to the severe carbohydrate restriction. Exercising at this point will also help in losing more weight. Note that the weight loss in the induction phase is more from water loss than fat. Reducing the carbohydrates result to losing water. Stored carbohydrates are at a ratio of ¾ water and ¼ carbohydrates. That is why it is very important to drink 2 liters or 8 glasses of water during the entire induction phase.

The induction phase may prove to be a bit difficult for most people. There may be decreased energy and other negative effects on the body. These can occur as the body adjusts and shifts from being carbohydrate dependent to a fat burner. Most dieters recommend eating once every 6 hours, eating 3 full meals or 5-6 small meals, and snacking. The cravings will be the hardest to address in this stage. Focus on eating more proteins and fat to combat the cravings. It helps to feel more satiated and full longer.

As you progress with the Atkins diet plan, the carbohydrate allowance is increased. The carbohydrate sources are from fiber-rich foods. Forget about eating white carbohydrates. Foods rich in white carbohydrates include white rice, anything made from white flour like pasta and bread, and white potatoes. At this point, fruits, vegetables, and foods with whole grains can be added. You are ready to move on to the next phase if you lost 15 pounds. If not, you may need to stay in the induction phase. Some people may need to stay in the induction phase for as long as 6 months.

The next phase in the Atkins diet program is the Ongoing Weight Loss phase or OWL. Daily carbohydrate intake is still markedly reduced compared with the US Dietary Allowance of 300 grams intake. The net carbohydrate allowance in the induction phase is increased each week by 5 net carbohydrate grams. The goal is to find the critical carbohydrate level for losing weight. Net carbohydrate intake is gradually increased per week, while observing if there is weight gain.

Example, if this week you increased carbohydrates by 5 grams and did not gain weight, it is OK. If you gained weight, go back to the previous net carbohydrate allowance. It is different with every individual. This phase lasts until the body weight is within 10 pounds or 4.5 kilograms of the desired weight. For the first week of the OWL phase, add small servings of the vegetables in the induction phase list. The next week, follow the developed carbohydrate ladder. This ladder consists of 9 rungs or steps and followed in exact order. Incorporate the allowed food items in small increments. The rungs actually consist of the food items that can be added to the previous meal plan. .

Gradual weight loss is maintained by a gradual transition from weight loss diet to weight maintenance. Carbohydrates are increased, only up to a point where the weight is maintained. This starts with the pre-maintenance phase. You are ready to enter this phase when your weight is 10 pounds or 4.5 kilograms away from the desired weight. The net carbohydrates in the meals are increased by 10 grams every week. The goal of this phase is to determine the critical carbohydrate level for weight maintenance. It refers to the maximum amount of carbohydrates that the dieter can consume in a day without adding weight. Usually, the amount is greater than that in the induction of the ketotic level. Hence, the dieter does not necessarily need to eat too little food for long. Observe your weight for the week after adding carbohydrates in the diet. If you gained weight or start to feel cravings, you may have too much carbohydrates in the meals. Return to the previous amounts.

At this phase, the dieter is allowed to eat the forbidden carbohydrates occasionally, at most, once a week. This is preparing the body for the lifetime maintenance phase. The body starts to lose the ketosis effect and protection. You can start eating starchy vegetables like sweet potatoes and whole grains (e.g., oatmeal). Do so in moderation. Continue drinking at least eight glasses of water. Increase the daily net carbohydrate intake by 10 grams every week, if you continue losing weight. If the dieter has achieved the desired weight, maintain it at that level for at least 6 months. After that, you can start adding 10 net grams again each week. Observe if you gain weight or not. Cut back if you gain weight.

Chapter 5 - atkins meal guide

The Atkins diet puts focus on the net carbohydrate content of each food. To help you determine the net carbohydrate, look for the total carbohydrate content in the label and that of fiber on the food label. Subtract the fiber content from the total carbohydrates. This will reflect as the net carbohydrates. If you are choosing unprocessed food, it may be more difficult to compute. Here is an example to for you to start counting those net carbohydrates.

For a 20-gram net carbohydrate per day:

· Cheese 3 oz (85 g) = 3g

· Eggs, 2 pieces = 1 g

· Mixed salad (3 cups, loosely heaped) = 3g

· Olives, 10 pieces = 2 g

· Cream, 1 Tablespoon = 0.5g

· Avocado, half = 2g

· Vegetable, cooked (1 cup) = 4g

· Sugar substitute, 2 teaspoon = 1g

· Lemon juice, 1 Tablespoon = 1.5g

· Salad dressing, 2 Tablespoon = 2g

Total net carbohydrate = 20g

Note that all these are to be eaten in one day, not in one meal. Cheeses are allowed at 3 to 4 oz a day. Types include Edam, mozzarella, cheddar, blue cheeses, and any cheese from goat, cow and sheep. Basically, for every 1 oz (28g) of cheese, it contains 1g of net carbohydrate. In a day, it is good to eat about 12 to 15 net carbohydrates of vegetables a day. These are high in vitamins and minerals, and are rich in fiber. These vegetables have 1g of net carbohydrates per cup:

· Fennel

· Lettuce: romaine, radicchio, rocket, endive, and all other types

· Cucumber

· Chive

· Alfalfa sprouts

· Celery

· Bok choy

· Chicory

· Mushrooms

· Radish

· Parsley

These other vegetables have higher net carbohydrate per cup (6g/cup) but add variety in the flavor.

· Asparagus

· Bamboo shoots

· Artichoke

· Brussels sprouts

· Broccoli

- Bean shoots

- Courgette

- Chard

- Cauliflower

- Cabbage

- Kale

- Leeks

- Onions

- Peppers

- Pumpkin

- Sauerkraut

- Okra

- Rhubarb

- Sugar snaps

- Squash

- String beans

- Turnips

- Tomatoes

Aside from the food listed above, you can add foods that do not contain carbohydrates like fish, fowl and meat. All fish are essentially carbohydrate free. You can add tuna, herring, sardines, salmon and trout to the list above. Fowl like duck, goose, quail, chicken, and turkey are good choices, too. Shellfish like oysters and mussels should be limited to 115g (4oz) per day because they do contain carbohydrates. Lobster, squids, prawns, and crabs are also allowed. All meats are permitted, like pork, beef, lamb, and veal.

To spice up your food, add herbs and spices like:

· cayenne pepper

· basil

· garlic

· dill

· coriander

· ginger

· rosemary

· oregano

· pepper

· thyme

· tarragon

· sage

To keep food more interesting, salad garnishes can be added like:

· sour cream

· sautéed mushroom

· grated cheese

· crisp bacon

· hardboiled egg

· dressings: oil, vinegar, lemon juice with herbs and spices

Hydration is very important. Drink plenty of water, at least 8 glasses of water each day. Allowed beverages include coffee, tea, and soda water. Clear broths or bouillon can also help curb cravings. Drink more water to combat cravings. Sometimes, these cravings are thirst in disguise.

For the Induction phase, avoid all fruits, brains, breads, dairy products (except butter and cheese), alcohol, and starchy vegetables. Strictly follow the 20g/day allocation of net carbohydrate intake. Eat more of proteins and fats. At each meal, eat at least 4-6 oz or 113-170 grams of protein, which is roughly equivalent to the size of two decks of cards. Do not hesitate to cook food with real butter, or add cream to your food. Enjoy eating foods that have fat in it. Choose food with monounsaturated and polyunsaturated fats. Avoid those that contain trans fat and saturated fats. Drink plenty of water. It will help with the cravings. Drink at least 8 glasses of water or 2 liters of water.

In phase 2 (Ongoing weight loss), whole foods are slowly added to the diet. These include nuts, yogurt and berries. The net carbohydrate daily intake is increased between 25 and 45 grams. You do not need to alter your induction phase meal plan. Increase the servings and you are good to go. The same food groups apply. If you are able to maintain weight loss, you are now ready to follow the 9 rungs of the carbohydrate ladder. It consists of the type of foods you are to gradually include in your diet. These are:

1. increase acceptable vegetables

2. Cheese

3. Nuts and seeds

4. Berries

5. Alcohol

6. Legumes

7. Other fruits

8.Starchy vegetables

9. Whole grains

When you are 10 pounds away from your desired weight, you are now ready to move on to phase 3. This is the pre-maintenance phase. More types of carbohydrates are added into your diet. The daily carbohydrate intake is increased by 10 grams per week. Check if you gain weight. Continue adding 10 grams per week until you find the amount of daily carbohydrates that will not result in weight gain. Carbohydrate sources that can be added are fruits, whole grains, and starchy vegetables. When you reach your target weight, maintain it for at least a month.

After which, you are now ready to enter the last phase. This is phase 4 of the Atkins diet, the lifetime maintenance phase. You are to maintain the determined daily net carbohydrate intake for the rest of your life.

Chapter 6 - the new atkins diet meal plan

Over the years, the Atkins diet had been subjected to controversies and criticisms. Particular controversial topic is the Atkins claim that one can lose weight while eating proteins, fats and rich foods like butter and full cream. Since the 70's, Atkins diet has been modified to address these criticisms. The program has recently been reformulated. The new Atkins diet has shifted from the original protein and fat diet advocate. Now, there is more focus on eating healthy and nutritionally dense foods. Portion control is also included in the new Atkins diet. Whole foods are given emphasis, too.

The common misconception about the Atkins diet is the food portion. It has been widely publicized and sensationalized that a dieter can eat unrestrained. As long as you keep away from the carbohydrates, you can eat as much as you want. This is not so. It has never been the case, according to the people behind the Atkins diet. The diet plan encourages eating proteins until one is satiated. There are no caloric restrictions or limits on the amount of proteins consumed. But that does not mean an eat-all-you-can fest the whole day. Eating proteins until satiated may raise eyebrows at first. The issue is overeating. In reality, protein intake has an internal control. It is self-limiting. In carbohydrates, it is very easy to keep munching on chocolate chip cookies the entire day and still want more. For proteins, it is unlikely to eat a pound of steak and still want more in just one meal.

Another misconception is on the difference between the induction phase and the rest of the diet program. In the induction phase, the net carbohydrates are counted, not the total. This is because the net carbohydrates are the only ones that have an impact on the body's blood sugar levels. Sugar alcohol carbohydrates and fiber do not affect blood sugar level, hence, are not counted. The induction phase requires a net carbohydrate intake of 20g (RDA is 300g).

In the original Atkins diet, all carbohydrates are treated and counted the same. The induction phase is only a stage that prepares the body to shift to fats as energy sources, and not heavily rely on carbohydrates. It is also where the body is said to be "cured" of the cravings for high carbohydrate foods like sweets. As the dieter progresses through the Atkins diet program, the carbohydrates are gradually increased until a certain level is reached. The goal of raising the carbohydrates gradually is to determine the state wherein there is neither weight loss nor weight gain. This can be within the USDA (US Dietary Allowance) standards, below or above. It all depends on the age, weight, and activity of the dieter.

The fat included in the Atkins diet is a major point of argument amongst diet experts. The Atkins program encourages eating fats to feel more satisfied with meals and delay hunger. It does not discriminate the type of fats incorporated in the diet. With the new Atkins diet plan, the fat must be of the healthy type. There is still no set limit to the amount of fat consumed. Choose lean protein sources that are low in carbohydrates. Incorporate fresh vegetables, fruits, and whole grain to the diet. Avoid processed foods. In contrast to the old Atkins diet, the new one is now putting emphasis on portion control. Before, you can all you want until you are satiated, as long as it is not carbohydrates. Now, the new Atkins program tells dieters to control the amount of food they consume.

There is a new emphasis placed on eating wholesome foods in the reformulated Atkins diet. Avoid unhealthy foods. These include sugar from candies, ice cream, soft drinks, and all others that use refined sugar. Artificial sweeteners are just as bad.

Watch out for food that used saccharin, aspartame, cyclamates, sucralose and acesulfame potassium.

Avoid highly processed food. They are generally unhealthy, whether you are trying to lose weight or not. While fats are essential in Atkins diet, stay away from hydrogenated or partially hydrogenated fats. Of course, never ever choose foods that have trans fat in it. Seed- and vegetable-oils that are high in omega-6 are also avoided. These include oils from cottonseed, grapeseed, corn, safflower, canola, soybean and sunflower. The most important foods to avoid and the ultimate no-no in Atkins diet are the white carbs. These foods are made with white flour (processed flour). Included also are the so-called gluten grains like wheat, barley and rye. White breads and pastas are rich in white carbohydrates. Avoid these as well. White rice and white potatoes are to be avoided, too.

Low carbohydrate food choices should be from real and unprocessed sources. These include fresh meats like lamb, pork, beef and chicken. Best are organic ones, or those that have been fed with grass. Fish caught in the wild are great low carbohydrate protein sources. Examples are salmon and trout. Pastured eggs and those that have been enriched with omega-3 are good to include in the daily meal. Fresh vegetables, fruits, and nuts are good additions to meals, or eaten as snacks. Fats are essential in the Atkins diet. Choose high-fat dairy products like yogurt, heavy cream, cheese and butter. Cod fish liver oil and olive oil can also be used.

Here is a sample menu plan and recipe when following the Atkins diet program. The numbers inside the parenthesis refer to the net carbohydrates contained in the food item.

· Breakfast:

2 scrambled eggs (1g)

Crack 2 eggs in a bowl. Add enough salt to taste. Add pepper for a little flavor. Whisk the eggs until well blended. Heat a pan and add about 1 tablespoon of oil. Use olive oil for a healthier alternative. Slowly pour the beaten eggs and fry until done. Remove.

2 oz. sautéed onions (1g)

In the same pan used to fry the eggs, add another tablespoon of oil. Chop a medium-sized onion. Sauté until it becomes translucent. Remove from the pan.

2 oz grated cheese (2g)

½ slice of avocado (2g)

Arrange the above ingredients. Place the sautéed onions on top of the eggs, then top with the grated cheese. Fold the egg over. Then serve with the avocado on the side. Drink allowable beverages. Better yet, drink water.

· Snack: grab a low carbohydrate power bar (2g)

· Lunch:

Grilled chicken

Get a 113g chicken breast. Season with salt and pepper. Heat a grill pan. Brush with some oil. When adequately hot, carefully place the chicken on the grill. Cook for about 2 minutes on each side or until cooked thoroughly. Set aside.

Mixed green salad

Mix together ½ cup of cherry tomatoes (2g), ½ cup cucumber slices (2g), 2 cups of mixed leaves (2g). Add a few chopped dill for flavor. Add 2 tablespoons of mayo for texture and richness. Drizzle with 2 tablespoons vinaigrette (2g).

- Snack: 1 celery stalk

- Dinner:

Grilled steak

Season an 8oz or 225g steak slice with salt and pepper. Grill to desired doneness.

Mixed salad

Mix together 1 cup rocket lettuce (1g) and ½ cup cucumber slices (1g). Top with 1 tablespoon ranch dressing (1g).

Notice that the above menu is very filling. You ate 3 complete meals with 2 snacks in one day. You did not deprive yourself of any of the food groups. Notice also that the total net carbohydrate consumed is only 19 grams, even below the drastic 20 grams in the induction phase. Great meal, isn't it?

Chapter 7 - atkins diet for life

The Atkins diet is also known as the Atkins Nutritional Approach. The program does not stop at achieving the desired weight. Rather, it helps to find the right amount of intake to maintain the desired weight. It continues for the rest of the dieter's life. The ultimate goal of the diet is to find the amount of carbohydrate intake that does not promote weight loss nor weight gain. Hence, you are being prepared to find the carbohydrate amount that your body needs for the day. This is called your ACE or Atkins Carbohydrate Equilibrium. Once achieved, it is now time to enter the last phase. This phase of the program helps you to turn this diet into a lifestyle. Good healthy food choices are encouraged throughout the program. This is to train you to be able to make adjustments in your food choices consciously and right off the bat. So that no matter what happens, wherever you are, you can reorient your eating habits to adhere to the ACE. If you have a high ACE or carbohydrate threshold, cautiously add new foods. If the new foods cause cravings, weight gain, or extreme hunger, remove them from your meals. If you have low carbohydrate threshold, stay away or limit your intake of whole grains and starchy vegetables.

At the lifetime maintenance phase, the body is already efficiently burning fat for energy. You can enjoy more fats in meals. Be aware of the type of fats you are eating, though. Make sure it is the healthy kind of fat. The idea is that the body is already burning fats and you can enjoy as much natural healthy fat as you want. No need to hold off the butter and olive oil in your salads and meal preparations. Add blue cheese and cream. Food will definitely be more interesting and flavorful.

Always keep in mind that you need to be aware of how your body responds to the food you eat. If a certain food item causes you to crave, or feel extremely hungry, it might be a good idea to avoid it for a while. Watch out for signs of carbohydrate intolerance with each food you eat. Dips in energy levels and weight gain might indicate avoidance of that food. Be vigilant of the carb creep. This is slowly letting in carbohydrates into the meals until you become dependent on them again. Early signs would be the cravings. Recheck your menu for any carbohydrate rich food. If a food cause you to crave, it is bad for you.

Apart from the weight loss, you can count the other benefits you have from the Atkins diet. This will encourage you to stick to the diet. Have blood laboratory checks and notice the improvement in your cholesterol levels. Take measurements of your waistline, hips, arms and legs. Chances are, you have lost a lot of inches in these areas. You will be able to fit into more clothes and show off your great new body. Take notice of the amount of energy you have for the rest of the day. Less energy drain and more energy to do the things you need to do. There is still spare energy to enjoy the things you love. With your high energy, you will also have better mood throughout the day.

Many people fall off the wagon after a few weeks. It is easy to get tired with the constant carbohydrate calculation. Menus may start to become boring. What is most disheartening is when the weighing scale shows no changes at all. While you do not gain weight, you also do not lose any. This is what is called the plateau stage. Most, if not all, dieters will experience this. So how do you pull yourself through this tough and challenging time? Here are 10 steps to push you on.

1. Realign your journey: Adjust your target weight loss rate to meet expectations. Do not set your goals that are too lofty and hard to reach.

2. Reassess your proteins: Maintain your protein intake to 6oz per meal.

3.Shift to counting calories: Try to monitor the amount of calories on your food plate. Look for food items that may be low in carbohydrates but very high in calories.

4.   Tally the net carbs: Keep a written record of the meals you take and manually count the net carbs. You might be overeating because of wrong estimation.

5.Add more vegetables: Consume 12 to 15 grams of net carbohydrates by eating vegetables allowed in the Atkins diet. Too few vegetables lead to constipation, which could increase weight readings.

6.   Reread labels: There may be hidden carbohydrates in commercially prepared sauce and condiments.

7.Control consumption of low-carb bars and shakes: They may be low-carb but still contain calories. It is easy to overeat on this stuff.

8.   Do not skip meals: Chances are, you will feel so hungry by the next meal. The result? It takes a longer time to feel full, hence, overeating.

9.   Check your medications: Consult your doctor about the medicines you are taking, if any. Some of these may be slowing down your weight loss.

10. Do not stress yourself: Stress stimulates cortisol production. This hormone increases the rate of fat storage, especially around the waist. Relax through yoga, exercise, and other stress management methods.

Be active. Engage in exercise, even if only for 20 minutes each day. It will reduce your risk for cardiovascular disease. It helps tone your body more, giving you a better look. Give and gain support to people who are also struggling with their weight. Keep yourself strong against sugary temptations. When going out or attending parties, it is good to snack on a celery stalk beforehand. Dip it in peanut butter. Chances are, you will be less hungry at the restaurant or party. You will less likely eat very tempting high-carbohydrates food on the menu.

Chapter 8: desserts recipes

Dark Mocha Pudding

Servings: 8 | Prep: 10 m | Style: American | Cook: 10 m

Ingredients

- 2 cups Organic Coconut Milk
- 1/2 cup Heavy Cream
- 1/8 tsp Salt
- 1/3 cup Erythritol Powder
- 3 tsps Sucralose Based Sweetener (Sugar Substitute)
- 2 large Egg Yolks
- 1 tsp dry Coffee (Instant Powder)
- 1 tbsp Cocoa Powder (Unsweetened)
- 1/2 tsp Thick-It-Up
- 1 tsp Vanilla Extract
- 2 oz Sugar Free Chocolate Chips
- 1 tbsp Unsalted Butter Stick

Directions

1. Place 1 3/4 cups of the coconut milk in a sauce pan with the heavy cream, salt and granular sugar substitutes. Bring to a simmer over medium heat.
2. While the milk is heating, whisk the egg yolks with the remaining 1/4 cup coconut milk and instant coffee. Once the milk mixture is hot pour a steady stream in the egg yolks while whisking to temper them. Once all the milk has been incorporated pour the mixture back into the sauce pan over medium heat. While it is heating back up, quickly whisk together the cocoa powder and Thick-It-Up in a small bowl

29

then whisk it into the milk and egg mixture. Cook and stir pudding continuously to be sure the egg does not curdle. Cook until it begins to thicken (mixture will still be slightly runny); about 2-3 minutes. Do not allow pudding to boil. Take off the heat once thickened; about 3-5 minutes.

3. Melt the chocolate with the butter in small bowl in a microwave at 30 second intervals. Do not overheat. Stir to blend and then scrape into the hot pudding stirring to blend completely. Remove from heat.

4. Cool quickly over an ice water bath; place plastic wrap on the surface to prevent a skin from forming. Once cooled place in the refrigerator to continue cooling or immediately dish into serving bowls, top with whipped cream if desired and serve. Makes 2 2/3 cups. Each serving is 1/3 cup. This pudding is very rich, consider serving it in a small glass dish layered with whipped cream.

Nutritional Information

- Protein : 3.3g
- Fat : 19g
- Fiber : 2g
- Calories :203

Decadent Chocolate Cake

Servings: 12 | Prep: 15 m | Style: American | Cook: 45 m

Ingredients

- 4 oz Unsweetened Baking Chocolate Squares
- 1/2 cup Unsalted Butter Stick
- 1 tbsp Tap Water
- 3/4 cup Sucralose Based Sweetener (Sugar Substitute)

- 2 tbsps Cocoa Powder (Unsweetened)
- 1 tsp Vanilla Extract
- 6 large Eggs (Whole)

Directions

1. Heat oven to 325°F. Grease an 8-inch spring form pan and line the bottom with parchment paper; grease paper and set aside.
2. Melt chocolate, butter and water in the top of a double boiler set over simmering water, stirring to combine. Remove from heat and transfer to a large bowl; cool to room temperature. Add ¼ cup of the sugar substitute, the cocoa powder and vanilla extract to chocolate mixture, stirring until combined.
3. In a medium bowl, with an electric mixer on medium-high, beat eggs until mixture forms thick ribbons when beater is lifted, about 6 minutes. Reduce speed to medium; gradually add remaining ½ cup sugar substitute and beat until combined, 1 minute. Stir one-third of the egg mixture into the chocolate mixture to lighten. In two additions, fold in remaining egg mixture until well combined.
4. Pour batter into prepared pan, smoothing top. Bake until evenly risen and almost set, 40-45 minutes (it will look like a brownie). Cool completely on a wire rack. To serve, run a knife around edge of pan and remove rim. Cut into 12 pieces and serve with whipped cream (optional).

Nutritional Information

- Protein : 4.5g
- Fat : 15g
- Fiber : 1.9g
- Calories :159

Decadent Chocolate Ice Cream

Servings: 8 | Prep: 240 m | Style: American | Cook: 20 m

Ingredients

- 2 large Egg Yolks
- 3 cups Heavy Cream
- 4 large Eggs (Whole)
- 3/4 cup Cocoa Powder (Unsweetened)
- 3/4 cup Sucralose Based Sweetener (Sugar Substitute)
- 1/4 tsp Salt
- 2 tsps Vanilla Extract
- 1/2 tsp Pure Almond Extract

Directions

1. Pour heavy cream into a heavy-bottomed 3-quart saucepan and place over medium heat. Allow to simmer but do not boil. Remove from heat and set aside.
2. In a large mixing bowl, combine the eggs, yolks, cocoa powder, sugar substitute and salt. With an electric mixer on medium, beat until thickened and smooth, 2 to 3 minutes, scraping sides of bowl with a rubber spatula. Using a ladle, remove about a cup of the hot cream from the pan, and gradually whisk into egg mixture (this tempers the eggs so they won't curdle). While whisking, pour tempered egg mixture into remaining cream in saucepan.
3. Place over medium heat and whisk until slightly thickened and coats the back of a wooden spoon; temperature should not go over 170°F.
4. Pour into a clean bowl, whisk in extracts and let stand until custard is cooled to room temperature, about 1 1/2 hours or place in a clean bowl set in a larger bowl filled with an ice water bath to chill quickly to room temperature. Refrigerate

2 hours, until well chilled, or cover with plastic wrap and refrigerate overnight to develop more flavor.
5. Freeze in ice cream maker according to manufacturers directions. When freezing process is complete, serve immediately for soft serve ice cream, or for firm ice cream, place in an airtight container and freeze 2 to 4 hours or overnight. (Can be stored in the freezer up to 1 month.) Makes about 1 quart; each serving = 1/2 cup. This recipe is acceptable in Phase 1; however the serving size would need to be decreased to 1/4 cup = 3.6g NC.

Nutritional Information

- Protein : 5.7g
- Fat : 36.7g
- Fiber : 2.7g
- Calories :373

Double Chocolate Cookies

Servings: 18 | Prep: 10 m | Style: American | Cook: 20 m

Ingredients

- 1/4 cup Unsalted Butter Stick
- 1/4 cup Xylitol
- 1 tsp Vanilla Extract
- 1 large Egg (Whole)
- 1 1/2 cups Blanched Almond Flour
- 2 tbsps Cocoa Powder (Unsweetened)
- 1/4 tsp Baking Soda
- 1/4 tsp Salt
- 3 packs Endulge Chocolate Candies

Directions

This recipe is suitable for all phases except for the first two weeks of Induction due to the nuts. Xylitol usually comes granulated but does not melt into the wet ingredients as well as regular sugar. For this reason be sure to measure the xylitol first and then powder it in a blender for 3-4 pulses. 1 cookie = 1 serving.

1. Preheat an oven to 350°F. Use a silpat mat or parchment paper on the cookie sheet.
2. Beat the softened butter with the powdered xylitol until light and fluffy; about 3 minues. Add the vanilla and egg and beat until combined.
3. Combine all the remaining dry ingredients except the candies, stir to blend and then add to the wet ingredients. Blend until fully incorporated then add the candies.
4. Form into 18 x 1-inch balls, spacing 1-inch apart and flatten slightly on the prepared cookie sheet. Bake for 10 minutes, remove from oven and allow to sit for 5 minutes then move to a cooling rack. Cookies may be stored in an airtight container at room temperature for up to 2 days.

Nutritional Information

- Protein : 2.7g
- Fat : 8.8g
- Fiber : 4.5g
- Calories :107

Earl Grey Tea and Chocolate Pots de Crème

Servings: 4 | Prep: 75 m | Style: French | Cook: 40 m

Ingredients

- 1 1/2 oz Unsweetened Baking Chocolate Squares
- 1 cup Heavy Cream
- 2/3 cup Tap Water
- 3 tea bags Tea Bags
- 4 large Egg Yolks
- 5 tbsps Sucralose Based Sweetener (Sugar Substitute)

Directions

1. Heat oven to 325°F. Place chocolate in a small bowl.
2. In a small saucepan over medium heat, bring cream and water to a simmer. Remove from heat.
3. Pour just enough cream mixture over chocolate to cover (about ½ cup). Add tea bags to remaining cream mixture in saucepan and let steep 10 minutes. Squeeze tea bags over mixture and remove.
4. Whisk chocolate mixture until smooth. Whisk egg yolks and sugar substitute into the warm cream mixture in saucepan until well mixed, then whisk in the chocolate until smooth. Pour mixture through a strainer into four 4-ounce ramekins or custard cups.
5. Place cups in a large roasting pan. Place roasting pan in oven and carefully pour boiling water into pan until water comes halfway up sides of cups. Cover entire pan with foil and bake 33-35 minutes, until custards are set but slightly jiggly in center.
6. Let stand in pan at room temperature 15 minutes. Remove cups, cover with plastic wrap (stretch wrap over edges of cup so wrap does not touch custard) and refrigerate until cold. Serve topped with a dollop of whipped cream, if desired.

Nutritional Information

- Protein : 5.3g
- Fat : 32.3g
- Fiber : 1.8g
- Calories :322

Endulge Chocolate Cups

Servings: 1 | Prep: 20 m | Style: American

Ingredients

- 1 1/2 oz Sugar Free Chocolate Chips

Directions

1. Line a muffin tin compartment with a paper cupcake liner. Place chocolate pieces in a Pyrex measuring cup. Microwave on 20 percent power for 30 seconds. Stir, and repeat process until pieces are melted but haven't completely lost their shape. Stir until smooth.
2. With a pastry brush, coat inside of cupcake liner with a layer of chocolate. Refrigerate 4 to 5 minutes, until chocolate sets. Repeat process until all the chocolate is used up. When chocolate is hardened, carefully peel off liner.
3. Cups may be made ahead, covered in plastic and stored in a cool place for up to 5 days.

Nutritional Information

- Protein : 1g
- Fat : 12.9g
- Fiber : 3g
- Calories :159

Endulgent Chocolate-Covered Strawberries

Servings: 24 | Prep: 25 m | Style: American

Ingredients

- 8 oz Sugar Free Chocolate Chips

- 24 large (1-3/8" dia) Strawberries

Directions

1. Line a baking sheet with aluminum foil or waxed paper. Break chocolate bars into pieces; place in the top part of a double boiler or a metal bowl set over (but not touching) a pot of simmering water. Stir one to two minutes, until chocolate is melted. Remove from heat.
2. Holding each strawberry by the stem, dip in chocolate, leaving a 1/4inch border at the top. Gently shake off excess chocolate; place berry on foil. Repeat with remaining berries. Reheat chocolate if necessary.
3. Chill berries 40 minutes, until chocolate is set. May be prepared up to a day ahead.

Nutritional Information

- Protein : 0.4g
- Fat : 3.1g
- Fiber : 1.1g
- Calories :44

Extra-Creamy Strawberry Shake

Servings: 2 | Prep: 5 m | Style: American

Ingredients

- 6 medium (1-1/4" dia) Strawberries
- 2 scoops Strawberry Whey Protein
- 1/2 cup Heavy Cream
- 1 tsp Vanilla Extract
- 2 cups Tap Water
- 2 individual packets Sucralose Based Sweetener (Sugar Substitute)

Directions

1. Place strawberries, protein mix, cream, vanilla, water, and sugar substitute in a blender and blend at high speed until very smooth.

Nutritional Information

- Protein : 23.5g
- Fat : 23.8g
- Fiber : 0.7g
- Calories :339

Firecracker Popsicles

Servings: 6 | Prep: 240 m | Style: American

Ingredients

- 1 cup Blueberries
- 1 cup Raspberries
- 1 cup Coconut Milk
- 6 tsps Xylitol
- 1/2 packet Stevia
- 1/2 tsp Coconut Extract

Directions

1. Puree the blueberries with 2 teaspoons xylitol and a pinch of stevia, set aside in a small bowl.
2. Puree the raspberries with 2 teaspoons xylitol and a pinch of stevia, set aside in a small bowl. If the raspberries are not very sweet add additional stevia to taste.

3. In a small bowl combine the coconut milk with 2 teaspoons xylitol, a pinch of stevia and 1/2 teaspoon of either coconut or vanilla extract.
4. Layer the popsicle mold: Start with the coconut milk, add 2-3 tablespoons then add a couple of tablespoons of each of the raspberry and blueberry purees, layering as you go. Once the popsicle is filled to about 1/2-inch from the top, take a knife, stick it in the center and gently swirl the knife to get the firecracker effect.
5. Freeze for at least 3 hours. May be kept frozen for up to 1 month. To release from the molds, run hot water over the molds until they slip off easily; about 5-10 seconds.

Nutritional Information

- Protein : 1.2g
- Fat : 8.3g
- Fiber : 5.9g
- Calories :110

Fresh Berry Tarts with Cream

Servings: 4 | Prep: 15 m | Style: American | Cook: 10 m

Ingredients

- 2/3 cup, slivered Almonds
- 1/2 cup Fresh Blueberries
- 1/4 cup Heavy Cream
- 1/2 cup Red Raspberries
- 2 tbsps Sucralose Based Sweetener (Sugar Substitute)

Directions

1. Heat broiler. Chop almonds and divide among 4 small ramekins. Sprinkle 1 tablespoon sugar substitute over the almonds. Place ramekins on a cookie sheet and broil until

the tops of the nuts are golden and the sugar substitute has melted. Remove and cool until at room temperature.

2. Whip the heavy cream and remaining tablespoon of sugar substitute until doubled in volume. Place one-quarter of blueberries and one-quarter of raspberries in each ramekin and top with a dollop of whipped cream. Serve immediately.

Nutritional Information

- Protein : 4.5g
- Fat : 14.6g
- Fiber : 3.6g
- Calories :177

Frozen Chocolate Fudge Tart

Servings: 12 | Prep: 210 m | Style: American | Cook: 20 m

Ingredients

- 5 tbsps Cocoa Powder (Unsweetened)
- 1/2 tsp Cinnamon
- 7 tbsps Sucralose Based Sweetener (Sugar Substitute)
- 4 tbsps Unsalted Butter Stick
- 3 oz Cream Cheese
- 4 oz Sugar Free Chocolate Chips
- 2 tsps Vanilla Extract
- 2 1/2 cups Heavy Cream
- 1 2/3 servings All Purpose Low-Carb Baking Mix
- 1 tsp dry Coffee (Instant Powder)

Directions

1. Preheat oven to 425°F.
2. For the crust: In a food processor, pulse the 1/2 cup baking mix, 4 tablespoons cocoa powder, cinnamon and 3 tablespoons granular sugar substitute to combine, about 10

seconds. Add cold chopped butter and pulse until mixture resembles a coarse meal, about 30 seconds. Add cream cheese and pulse until mixture begins to come together, about 30 more seconds.

3. Transfer dough to a 9-inch pie plate and pat into an even layer on bottom and sides. Prick the dough about 15 times with a fork and crimp edges decoratively. Cover lightly with aluminum foil and bake 10 minutes, until set. Uncover and bake 10 more minutes until light golden brown. Cool crust before filling.

4. For the filling: Place chocolate and 1 teaspoon vanilla extract in a medium bowl. Heat one cup cream and instant coffee over medium-high heat until just about to boil, about 4 minutes. Pour over chocolate, let stand 3 minutes, then stir until chocolate is melted. Pour into pie shell, smooth top and chill 30 minutes.

5. In a medium bowl with an electric mixer on high speed, beat remaining cream, 4 tablespoons sugar substitute, 1 teaspoon vanilla extract and 1 tablespoon cocoa powder until medium peaks form, about 4 minutes. Spread over chocolate layer and freeze at least 2.5 hours or until firm. Remove from freezer 10 minutes before serving.

Nutritional Information

- Protein : 6.1g
- Fat : 28.7g
- Fiber : 1.9g
- Calories :303

Frozen Peanut Butter Chocolate Cheesecake Bombs

Servings: 12 | Prep: 60 m | Style: American

Ingredients

- 6 oz Cream Cheese
- 1/3 cup Natural Creamy Peanut Butter 1/3 Less Sodium & Sugar
- 2 tbsps Xylitol
- 1 tsp Vanilla Extract
- 1 pinch Stevia
- 1 cup Heavy Cream
- 1/8 tbsp Xanthan Gum
- 3 bars Snack Caramel Double Chocolate Crunch Bar

Directions

1. Powder the xylitol before using. To do this place 2 tablespoons in a blender and pulse 3-4 times until powdered.
2. Beat softened cream cheese with a mixer on medium speed until creamy. Add peanut butter, powdered granular sugar substitute, and vanilla; beat to combine. Taste and increase sweetness if desired by adding a pinch of stevia.
3. Add 1 cup cream and 1/4 teaspoon xanthan gum (optional, helps decreases ice crystal formation when frozen); beating until light and fluffy.
4. Cut Atkins bars lengthwise into three segments then finely chop the segments; fold into mixture. Using a 2 tablespoon scoop or measure drop onto a wax paper covered baking sheet (small enough to fit in your freezer or use a silicon mold filling each with 2 Tbsp). Place in the freezer until fully frozen; at least 4 hours. To serve, eat directly from the freezer or place 2 on a serving plate and allow to partially thaw in the refrigerator for 30 minutes. The recipe makes 24 bombs. Each serving is 2 bombs (or 4 Tbsp total).

Nutritional Information

- Protein : 5.2g
- Fat : 18.3g
- Fiber : 5.3g
- Calories :208

Frozen Peppermint Pie

Servings: 8 | Prep: 20 m | Style: American

Ingredients

- 1 cup Heavy Cream
- 6 pieces Sugar Free Starlite Mints
- 1 tbsp Organic Virgin Coconut Oil
- 1/2 cup Almond Meal Flour
- 5 servings Atkins Snack Dark Chocolate Decadence Bar
- 8 servings Easy Peppermint Ice Cream

Directions

Use the Atkins recipe to make Easy Peppermint Ice Cream; you will need 1 full recipe (about 3 cups). Please note, you can use vanilla sugar free ice cream instead of the Easy Peppermint Ice Cream but it will add about 5g NC to each serving. If you choose to do this you will need 12 mints (crushed) - add half of them to the ice cream mixture and the other half to the top.

1. Allow the ice cream to sit at room temperature for about 20 minutes to soften.
2. Chop the Atkins Dark Chocolate Decadence bar into 1 inch pieces. Place in a food processor and process until it resembles fine crumbs. Add the coconut oil and almond meal and process until combined. Press into a pie place and place in the freezer while preparing the rest of the filling.
3. Whip heavy cream to firm peaks. Fold together the softened ice cream with the whipped cream and pour into the prepared pie shell. Sprinkle crushed peppermint candies on the top and place in the freezer until fully set (about 1 hour).

Nutritional Information

- Protein : 9.6g
- Fat : 55.2g
- Fiber : 15.7g
- Calories :629

Ginger Flan

Servings: 6 | Prep: 180 m | Style: French | Cook: 25 m

Ingredients

- 3 large Egg Yolks
- 2 large Eggs (Whole)
- 1 1/2 cups Heavy Cream
- 1 cup Tap Water
- 8 individual packets Sucralose Based Sweetener (Sugar Substitute)
- 1 tsp Vanilla Extract
- 3 tsps Ginger

Directions

1. Heat oven to 350°F. Place a roasting pan on center shelf in oven and fill almost half way with boiling water.
2. In a blender, combine egg yolks and whole eggs, cream, water, sugar substitute, vanilla, and ginger until very smooth.
3. Pour through a sieve into a shallow 1-quart baking dish. Carefully place dish in roasting pan (water should come up halfway up sides). Bake 30-35 minutes until a knife inserted in center comes out clean.
4. Transfer to wire rack; cool to room temperature. Spray a piece of plastic wrap with cooking spray, lay directly over flan and chill 3 hours in refrigerator.

5. Remove plastic wrap and un-mold by placing a platter or plate over the top and inverting the platter onto a table so that the pan is now upside down on the platter. Remove top pan.

Nutritional Information

- Protein : 4.6g
- Fat : 26g
- Fiber : 0g
- Calories :265

Ginger Ice Cream with Caramelized Pears

Servings: 10 | Prep: 180 m | Style: American | Cook: 10 m

Ingredients

- 1 small (approx 3 per lb) Pear
- 3 1/2 cups Heavy Cream
- 1/2 cup Tap Water
- 1/4 cup slices (1" dia) Ginger
- 7 large Egg Yolks
- 2 tsps Unsalted Butter Stick
- 4 tbsps Sugar Free Vanilla Syrup
- 2/3 cup Sucralose Based Sweetener (Sugar Substitute)

Directions

1. Combine cream, water and ginger in a heavy, medium saucepan over medium heat. Bring almost to a boil; remove from the heat and let stand 10 minutes.
2. Whisk egg yolks and sugar substitute in a large bowl until lightened and thick. Gradually whisk half of the hot cream into egg mixture; return mixture to pan. Cook, stirring

constantly, over medium heat until mixture registers 170°F on an instant-read thermometer or is thick enough to coat the back of a spoon.

3. Strain through a fine-mesh strainer into an airtight container, pressing with a spoon to extract liquid from ginger solids. Cover and refrigerate until cold. Pour mixture into ice cream maker and churn according to manufacturer's instructions.

4. Transfer to an airtight container and freeze until ready to serve. Just before serving, melt butter in a small skillet over high heat; add pear and cook until tender and lightly browned, 3 to 4 minutes. Pour syrup into a small serving bowl; stir pear into syrup. Scoop ice cream into bowls; top with pears.

Nutritional Information

- Protein : 3.7g
- Fat : 35g
- Fiber : 0.5g
- Calories :351

Holiday Cookies

Servings: 24 | Prep: 25 m | Style: American | Cook: 12 m

Ingredients

- 1 cup Whole Grain Soy Flour
- 3 tsps Baking Soda
- 3 tbsps Sucralose Based Sweetener (Sugar Substitute)
- 4 oz Cream Cheese
- 2 tbsps Unsalted Butter Stick
- 2 tbsps Sour Cream (Cultured)
- 1 large Egg (Whole)
- 1 tsp Vanilla Extract

Directions

1. Preheat oven to 350°F. Line a baking sheet with parchment paper and set aside.
2. In a food processor, pulse soy flour, baking soda, sugar substitute, cream cheese and butter for 30 seconds, until texture resembles a coarse meal.
3. In a small bowl, mix together sour cream, egg and vanilla extract. Add sour cream mixture to soy mix mixture and pulse until just-combined, about 15 seconds. Chill in freezer 10 minutes or until firm.
4. Roll dough out between 2 sheets of plastic wrap or waxed paper to 1/8 thickness. Using cookie cutters, cut out dough in desired shapes. Arrange cookies on prepared baking sheet and bake cookies 10-12 minutes, until lightly golden. Allow to cool completely before decorating.

Nutritional Information

- Protein : 1.8g
- Fat : 3.7g
- Fiber : 0.3g
- Calories :46

Indulgent Espresso Chocolate Cake

Servings: 8 | Prep: 25 m | Style: American | Cook: 35 m

Ingredients

- 10 oz Sugar Free Chocolate Chips
- 10 tbsps Unsalted Butter Stick
- 1 tsp rounded Coffee (Instant Powder, Decaffeinated)
- 1 tbsp Tap Water
- 1 tsp Vanilla Extract
- 1/4 tsp Salt

- 24 tsps Erythritol
- 1 pinch Stevia
- 4 large Eggs (Whole)
- 1/3 cup Cocoa Powder (Unsweetened)

Directions

1. Preheat oven to 325°F. Grease an 8-inch round baking pan and line with parchment paper (a spring form pan works best). Set aside.
2. Melt chocolate and butter in a double boiler. Remove from heat and transfer to a large bowl. Alternatively melt chocolate with butter in a small bowl in the microwave at 30 second intervals; stirring in between. In a small cup, mix espresso powder, water, vanilla and salt; stir into chocolate. Set mixture aside to cool.
3. With an electric mixer on medium-high speed, beat eggs, 1/2 cup (24 tsp) granular sugar substitute, stevia and cocoa powder until it falls in thick ribbons when the beater is lifted, about 6 minutes. In three additions, fold eggs into the chocolate mixture.
4. Pour batter into prepared pan and smooth top. Bake 30-35 minutes, or until a toothpick inserted near middle of cake comes out with a few moist crumbs and cake is evenly raised. Cool completely on a wire rack. To remove cake, run a knife around edge of pan. Dip bottom of pan into hot water for 1 minute, then turn cake out onto cutting board. (if using a spring form pan, carefully remove sides and serve on the platter.) Turn right side up onto a serving platter. Serve with whipped cream and raspberries (Phase 2 or Atkins 40 only), if desired.

Nutritional Information

- Protein : 4.8g
- Fat : 28.7g
- Fiber : 3.9g
- Calories :314

Irish Coffee

Servings: 6 | Prep: 5 m | Style: Other | Cook: 10 m

Ingredients

- 36 fl ozs Decaffeinated Coffee
- 3 tsps Sucralose Based Sweetener (Sugar Substitute)
- 9 fl oz (no ice) Whiskey
- 1/2 cup Heavy Cream

Directions

1. In a small saucepan, warm whiskey over medium-low heat (do not boil). Stir sugar substitute and whiskey into brewed coffee.
2. In the small bowl of an electric mixer, beat heavy cream on medium to soft peaks.
3. Divide coffee among 6 cups, and top each with a dollop of whipped cream.

Nutritional Information

- Protein : 0.6g
- Fat : 7.4g
- Fiber : 0g
- Calories :168

Lemon Mousse

Servings: 8 | Prep: 180 m | Style: French | Cook: 20 m

Ingredients

- 1 package (1 oz) Gelatin Powder (Unsweetened)

- 1/4 cup Fresh Lemon Juice
- 7 large Eggs (Whole)
- 6 individual packets Sucralose Based Sweetener (Sugar Substitute)
- 1 1/2 fl oz (no ice) Brandy
- 1 1/2 cups Heavy Cream

Directions

1. For this recipe substitute Grand Marnier or orange liquor for the brandy to give it more citrus flavor. If you prefer not to consume uncooked egg whites, use a powdered egg white product (sold in the baking section of most supermarkets) instead.
2. In a medium bowl, dissolve gelatin in lemon juice. Set bowl over a saucepan of simmering water (water should not touch the bottom of the bowl). Separate the whites from the yolks; place the whites in a large bowl and place the yolks into a sauce pan.
3. Whisk together the egg yolks and sugar substitute. Cook while whisking constantly over medium-high heat until a candy thermometer registers 170°F (about 4 minutes). Remove from heat; stir in brandy or orange liqueur. Transfer to a large bowl.
4. With an electric beater, beat egg whites until stiff peaks form; set aside. In another large bowl whip the cream until stiff peaks form. Fold egg whites into yolk-gelatin mixture until combined. Gently fold in whipped cream. Taste for sweetness; adjust if necessary. Cover with foil and refrigerate until well chilled.

Nutritional Information

- Protein : 7g
- Fat : 20.6g
- Fiber : 0g
- Calories :236

Low Carb Pumpkin Pecan Cheesecake

Servings: 10 | Prep: 25 m | Style: Other | Cook: 50 m

Ingredients

- 1 1/2 cup halves Pecan Nuts
- 1 tbsp Sucralose Based Sweetener (Sugar Substitute)
- 1/2 tsp Cinnamon
- 2 tbsps Unsalted Butter Stick
- 1 large Egg White
- 24 oz Cream Cheese
- 1 cup Heavy Cream
- 2/3 cup Sucralose Based Sweetener (Sugar Substitute)
- 15 oz Pumpkin (Without Salt, Canned)
- 1 tsp Vanilla Extract
- 1 tsp Pumpkin Pie Spice
- 3 large Eggs (Whole)

Directions

To make crust:

1. Heat oven to 350°F.
2. In a food processor, combine pecans, 1 tablespoon sugar substitute and cinnamon. Process until finely ground. Add the butter (melted) and egg white and pulse a few times to combine; press onto the bottom of a 9-inch springform pan, rounding up to cover the pan seam. Bake until golden and set, 8 to 10 minutes. Cool completely on a wire rack.

To make filling:

1. Reduce oven to 325°F.
2. Combine cream cheese, 2/3 cup sugar substitute and cream in a large bowl. With an electric mixer at medium speed,

beat until smooth. Add pumpkin purée, vanilla and pumpkin pie spice, mixing to combine. Beat in eggs, one at a time, just until combined.

3. Pour batter over crust. Bake until just set, 45 to 50 minutes. Turn off oven and let stand 10 minutes; transfer to a wire rack and cool completely.
4. Cover and refrigerate until chilled, 4 hours or overnight. Slice and serve.

Nutritional Information

- Protein : 8.6g
- Fat : 46.7g
- Fiber : 2.8g
- Calories :485

Low-Carb Chocolate Blueberry Cheesecake Tartlets

Servings: 12 | Prep: 360 m | Style: American | Cook: 40 m

Ingredients

- 2 cups Almond Meal Flour
- 4 tbsps Cocoa Powder (Unsweetened)
- 1 tbsp Sucralose Based Sweetener (Sugar Substitute)
- 1/4 cup Unsalted Butter Stick
- 6 oz Cream Cheese
- 1/2 cup Ricotta Cheese (Whole Milk)
- 2 large Eggs (Whole)
- 1/2 tsp Vanilla Extract
- 1/2 cup Sucralose Based Sweetener (Sugar Substitute)
- 1 cup Fresh Blueberries
- 1 tbsp Tap Water
- 1 large Egg Yolk

Directions

1. Preheat oven to 350°F. Liberally grease the cups of a 12-cup muffin tin, or 2 x 12 mini muffin pans or use muffin papers. In a medium bowl, whisk together almond meal, 3 tablespoons cocoa powder, and Splenda. Pour in butter and stir with fork until it forms coarse crumbs. Place one heaping tablespoon of almond crust into the bottom of each mini muffin tin or about 2 1/2 tablespoons in the regular muffin tin wells or paper cups. Using your fingers, press gently to work dough down and up the sides of the tin. Repeat until all muffin tins are filled. Place pan in oven and bake 5-7 minutes. Remove from oven and let cool.

2. Place cream cheese, ricotta cheese, eggs, vanilla, 1 tablespoon cocoa powder, and Splenda into a blender, and puree until smooth and free of lumps. Pour cream cheese mixture evenly into cooled crusts, leaving 1/4-inch rim of space at the top of each cup. Place pan back in oven and bake for 30-35 minutes for large muffin tins or 10-12 minutes for mini muffin tins, until the batter is no longer wet and firms around the edges. Remove from heat and let cool to room temperature.

3. Prepare the topping. In a small saucepan, add blueberries and water over medium heat. Bring to simmer, mashing blueberries with the back of a wooden spoon, until blueberries are hot and have released their juices. Place your egg yolk in a small bowl. Whisking swiftly and continuously, add a tablespoon of warm blueberry juice to yolks to temper. Repeat again two more times until yolk is tempered. Whisking quickly and constantly, pour tempered yolk into pan with blueberries. Stir, cooking, until blueberries are significantly thickened. Remove from heat and let cool slightly. Set aside to cool.

4. Spoon blueberry topping evenly over the tops of the cheesecake cups, spreading to cover evenly. Place muffin tin in refrigerator and let cool 4-5 hours or overnight, until

chilled completely. To serve, carefully pop cheesecake cups out of muffin tin and place on serving tray. Two per person if using the mini muffin tins or 1 per person if using the regular muffin tins.

Nutritional Information

- Protein : 7.8g
- Fat : 20.8g
- Fiber : 2.9g
- Calories :240

Mascarpone Parfait

Servings: 4 | Prep: 15 m | Style: Italian

Ingredients

- 1 cup Heavy Cream
- 8 oz Mascarpone
- 1 tbsp Sucralose Based Sweetener (Sugar Substitute)

Directions

1. In the large bowl of an electric mixer, beat heavy cream on medium-high to soft peaks.
2. Reduce speed to medium; add mascarpone and sugar substitute, beating just until smooth, 15 to 30 seconds. Divide and spoon the cream mixture into four parfait cups.
3. Garnish with mint sprigs and lemon peel, if desired.

Nutritional Information

- Protein : 5.3g
- Fat : 48.5g
- Fiber : 0g
- Calories :451

Mexican Hot Chocolate Souffle

Servings: 2 | Prep: 15 m | Style: French | Cook: 17 m

Ingredients

- 1 tsp Unsalted Butter Stick
- 9 tsps Erythritol
- 4 tbsps Sugar Free Chocolate Chips
- 2 large Egg Yolks
- 1/2 fl oz Tap Water
- 1 tsp Vanilla Extract
- 3/4 tsp Cinnamon
- 1/8 tbsp Red or Cayenne Pepper
- 3 large Egg Whites
- 1 pinch Stevia

Directions

1. Preheat oven to 400°F. Grease the bottom and up the sides of a 2-cup deep souffle dish with butter and sprinkle 1 1/2 teaspoons granular sugar substitute (erythritol) to coat all buttered areas. Set aside.
2. Melt the chocolate in a small bowl in a microwave at 30 second intervals until melted through. Do not overheat and stir between intervals.
3. In a medium bowl whisk 2 egg yolks with 1 tablespoon warm water, 1 teaspoon vanilla, 3/4 teaspoon ground cinnamon and 1/8 teaspoon cayenne pepper (add more if more spice is desired). Add the melted chocolate and whisk until incorporated and smooth. Set aside.
4. In a medium bowl whip the egg whites with 2 1/2 tablespoons granular sugar substitute (erythritol) and a large pinch of stevia to stiff peaks. Whisk a few tablespoons of the egg whites into the chocolate mixture, then quickly but gently fold in the remaining egg whites until a lighter airy

mixture results and all ingredients are blended (do not over blend or you will deflate the egg whites).

5. Pour into the souffle dish and bake on a sheet pan for 15-18 minutes. The souffle will rise over the top of the dish and it should appear slightly jiggly but not wet in the center when shaken. Serve immediately.

Nutritional Information

- Protein : 8.9g
- Fat : 15.8g
- Fiber : 2.7g
- Calories :4220

Mixed Berry Shortcakes

Servings: 6 | Prep: 35 m | Style: Other | Cook: 15 m

Ingredients

- 1 cup Whole Grain Soy Flour
- 1 tsp Baking Powder (Straight Phosphate, Double Acting)
- 2 2/3 tbsps Sucralose Based Sweetener (Sugar Substitute)
- 1 tsp Salt
- 6 tbsps Unsalted Butter Stick
- 1 2/3 cups Heavy Cream
- 1/4 cup Sour Cream (Cultured)
- 1 cup whole Strawberries
- 1 large Egg (Whole)
- 1 cup Blueberries
- 1 cup Raspberries
- 1/2 cup half Pecans

Directions

1. Preheat oven to 375°F.

2. In a food processor, pulse flour, baking powder, pecans, 3 tablespoons of the sugar substitute and salt until nuts are finely ground. (If you don't have a food processor, grind the nuts in a nut or coffee grinder.)
3. Add the butter and pulse until its the texture of cornmeal. In a liquid measuring cup or bowl, whisk 2/3 cup of the heavy cream, sour cream and egg. Pour evenly over the dry mixture and pulse just until combined.
4. Chill dough for 30 minutes. Separate dough into 12 equal-sized pieces (you'll need about 3 1/2 tablespoons of dough for each piece). Put each piece into a disk measuring 2 1/2 to 3-inches across. Space disks evenly on baking sheet, leaving 1 inch between biscuits to allow for spreading during the baking process.
5. Bake shortcakes about 20 minutes, until bottoms are golden brown. Cool on baking sheet set on a wire rack.
6. With an electric mixer on medium speed, beat remaining cup of heavy cream with remaining 2 teaspoons sugar substitute until soft peaks form.
7. To assemble: Dollop 1/4 cup whipped cream on 6 six shortcakes, top with 1/2 cup berries and cover with remaining shortcakes.

Nutritional Information

- Protein : 8.8g
- Fat : 47.6g
- Fiber : 4.5g
- Calories :512

Mocha Granita

Servings: 6 | Prep: 195 m | Style: Other

Ingredients

- 1 cup Tap Water
- 1 cup (8 fl oz) Coffee (Brewed From Grounds)
- 10 individual packets Sucralose Based Sweetener (Sugar Substitute)
- 1/3 cup Cocoa Powder (Unsweetened)
- 4 tbsps Sugar Free Chocolate Syrup

Directions

1. Mix water, coffee, and sugar substitute in a heavy saucepan over medium heat. Whisk in cocoa powder and syrup. Bring mixture to a gentle boil.
2. Simmer, stirring constantly, 3 minutes. Remove from heat; pour mixture through a fine strainer into a large measuring cup. Refrigerate until cold.
3. Pour mixture into ice cube trays, filling only half way. Freeze until firm. Before serving, process chocolate cubes in a food processor until chopped and slushy.
4. Serve immediately.

Nutritional Information

- Protein : 1.1g
- Fat : 0.7g
- Fiber : 1.8g
- Calories :20

Mocha-Hazelnut Ice Cream

Servings: 12 | Prep: 255 m | Style: Other | Cook: 18 m

Ingredients

- 3 1/2 cups Heavy Cream
- 3 oz Unsweetened Baking Chocolate Squares

- 1/3 cup Cocoa Powder (Unsweetened)
- 3 tsp roundeds Coffee (Instant Powder, Decaffeinated)
- 6 large Egg Yolks
- 1 cup Sucralose Based Sweetener (Sugar Substitute)
- 1 tbsp Vanilla Extract
- 1/3 cup chopped Hazelnuts or Filberts

Directions

1. In a medium saucepan, combine 3 cups of the cream, chocolate, cocoa powder and coffee granules; cook over medium-low heat, stirring occasionally, until chocolate melts and mixture just begins to simmer. Remove from heat and cool to room temperature. Whisk until smooth.
2. In a medium bowl, whisk egg yolks, remaining 1/2 cup cream and sugar substitute together until blended. Gradually whisk 1 cup of chocolate mixture into yolk mixture; add to saucepan with remaining chocolate mixture and whisk to combine.
3. Cook over medium-low heat, stirring constantly, until mixture coats the back of a spoon (175°F on a candy thermometer), about 3 minutes. Remove from heat; stir in vanilla and cool slightly.
4. Pour custard into a glass or metal bowl; cover with plastic wrap and refrigerate for 4 hours or overnight. Pour custard into ice-cream maker; freeze according to manufacturers directions.
5. During last 5 minutes, add hazelnuts. Transfer to an airtight container, cover and freeze for 4 hours or overnight. Let stand at room temperature until soft enough to scoop, about 15 minutes.

Nutritional Information

- Protein : 4.7g
- Fat : 34.1g
- Fiber : 2.3g
- Calories :341

Molten Chocolate Cake

Servings: 4 | Prep: 5 m | Style: American | Cook: 8 m

Ingredients

- 6 tbsps Unsalted Butter Stick
- 2 oz Baking Chocolate Squares
- 2 large Egg Yolks
- 1 tbsp Whole Grain Soy Flour
- 2 large Eggs (Whole)
- 1/3 cup Sucralose Based Sweetener (Sugar Substitute)
- 1 tsp Vanilla Extract

Directions

1. Preheat oven to 375°F.
2. Generously grease four 6-ounce custard cups with butter and dust with sugar substitute. Place cups on a baking sheet.
3. Place butter and chocolate in a double boiler over medium heat and cook until just melted, about 3 minutes (or 1 minute in a microwave on high). Remove from heat and let cool to room temperature.
4. Pour chocolate mixture into a large bowl; add soy flour and stir until just combined. Set aside.
5. In a large bowl, beat eggs, egg yolks, sugar substitute and vanilla with an electric mixer on high speed until almost firm peaks form, about 4 minutes.
6. In three additions, fold egg mixture into chocolate mixture.
7. Divide batter in cups. Bake 8 -9 minutes until a toothpick inserted near edge comes out clean and inserted in center comes out with some batter.

8. Cool 3 minutes. Run knife around edge, turn upside down to release onto serving plates. Serve immediately. Makes 4 servings.

Nutritional Information

- Protein : 6g
- Fat : 29.1g
- Fiber : 2.2g
- Calories :302

Old Fashioned Bread Pudding

Servings: 6 | Prep: 40 m | Style: Other | Cook: 60 m

Ingredients

- 1/2 cup Sucralose Based Sweetener (Sugar Substitute)
- 1 cup Heavy Cream
- 1 cup Tap Water
- 6 large Eggs (Whole)
- 1 tsp Vanilla Extract
- 1 tsp Cinnamon
- 8 servings Atkins Cuisine Bread

Directions

1. If you have a vanilla bean, use the seeds scraped from 1 whole bean. Instead of 1 teaspoon cinnamon substitute 1 3-inch cinnamon stick.
2. Preheat oven to 350°F. Generously butter a 9x9 -inch baking pan; set aside.
3. In a large bowl, whisk together eggs and sugar substitute.

4. In a medium saucepan over medium heat, bring cream, water, vanilla and cinnamon to a boil. Slowly whisk hot cream mixture into egg mixture. Add bread and toss well. Let stand 10 minutes, turning occasionally with a rubber spatula.
5. Transfer pudding mixture into to prepared pan. Place pan in a larger roasting pan, fill the outer pan with enough hot water to come half way up the sides of the pudding pan.
6. Bake for until set, about 55 minutes. Let cool for 15 minutes before cutting. Serve warm or chilled. Makes 6 servings.

Nutritional Information

- Protein : 14.2g
- Fat : 23.5g
- Fiber : 2.4g
- Calories :297

Panna Cotta

Servings: 6 | Prep: 195 m | Style: Italian | Cook: 5 m

Ingredients

- 1 package (1 oz) Gelatin Powder (Unsweetened)
- 2 cups Heavy Cream
- 8 individual packets Sucralose Based Sweetener (Sugar Substitute)
- 1 tsp Vanilla Extract

Directions

1. Lightly oil 6 6-ounce custard cups. In small bowl sprinkle gelatin over 3 tablespoons cold water, let sit 5 minutes until softened.
2. Meanwhile, in medium saucepan combine heavy cream, 1/2 cup water, sugar substitute and scrapped out vanilla bean seeds or use vanilla extract. Bring to a boil over medium heat.

3. Remove from heat, add gelatin mixture; stir until melted. Pour mixture into prepared cups. Cover surface with plastic wrap to prevent skin from forming. Refrigerate at least 3 hours.
4. Turn out onto serving plates.

Nutritional Information

- Protein : 2.6g
- Fat : 29.6g
- Fiber : 0g
- Calories :287

Passover Angel Food Cake with Rhubarb-Strawberry Sauce

Servings: 12 | Prep: 120 m | Style: Italian | Cook: 30 m

Ingredients

- 1 cup Matzo Meal
- 1 1/2 cups Sucralose Based Sweetener (Sugar Substitute)
- 1/2 tsp Salt
- 1 3/4 large Egg Whites
- 2 tsps Vanilla Extract
- 1/2 tsp Pure Almond Extract
- 12 oz Rhubarb
- 1 cup half Strawberries

Directions

For the cake: Heat oven to 375°F.

1. In a bowl, whisk cake meal, 1 1/4 cup sugar substitute and salt to combine. Place mixture in a wire sieve set over the

bowl. With an electric mixer on medium, beat egg whites until stiff peaks form. Stir in extracts.

2. In three additions, sift dry ingredients over the whites, gently folding in with a rubber spatula. Transfer batter to a 10 tube pan.
3. Bake 30 minutes, until cake begins to pull away from the sides of the pan. Invert cake in pan over a funnel or bottle neck, if pan does not have feet. Cool completely, about 1 1/2 hours.
4. With narrow spatula or knife, loosen cake from sides of pan and gently shake onto serving plate.

For the sauce:

1. In a medium pot, mix rhubarb, 1/2 cup strawberries, 1/4 cup sugar substitute and 1/4 cup water. Cook over medium heat 15 minutes, until rhubarb falls apart. Reduce heat and stir frequently during the last 5 minutes of cooking time.
2. Remove from heat; transfer to a bowl and fold in remaining strawberries. Cool completely and serve with cake. Makes 12 servings.

Nutritional Information

*   Protein : 5.2g
*   Fat : 0.2g
*   Fiber : 1.1g
*   Calories :80

Peach-Buttermilk Sherbert

Servings: 8 | Prep: 1440 m | Style: American | Cook: 20 m

Ingredients

*   3 medium (2-1/2" dia) (approx 4 per lb) Peaches
*   1/2 cup Xylitol

- 1 pinch Stevia
- 1/4 cup Fresh Lemon Juice
- 1/2 tsp Salt
- 1 cup Buttermilk (Reduced Fat, Cultured)
- 1 cup Heavy Cream

Directions

1. Coarsely dice peaches. In a medium pan combine the peaches and granular sugar substitutes; cook over medium heat for 15-20 minutes until very soft. Remove from heat and allow to cool for 10 minutes.
2. In a blender puree the peaches and cooking juices with lemon juice and salt (adjust to your taste). Add the buttermilk and cream. Mix to combine and place in the refrigerator overnight or at least 4 hours to chill.
3. Place the mixture in an ice cream maker and follow manufacturers directions. Once the sherbert is done serve immediately or pack into a freezer-safe container and place in freezer. This sherbert will keep in the freezer for up to one month. Place frozen sherbert in the refrigerator for 20-30 minutes before serving and use an ice cream scoop that has been dipped in hot water to serve more easily. Makes 1 quart; 1 serving = 1/2 cup.

Nutritional Information

- Protein : 2g
- Fat : 12.3g
- Fiber : 12.8g
- Calories :177

Peanut Butter and Jelly Thumbprints

Servings: 18 | Prep: 5 m | Style: American | Cook: 20 m

Ingredients

- 1 cup Natural Creamy Peanut Butter 1/3 Less Sodium & Sugar
- 24 tsps Erythritol
- 1 large Egg (Whole)
- 1 tsp Vanilla Extract
- 1/2 tsp Baking Soda
- 1/2 tsp Salt
- 6 tbsps Sugar Free Seedless Blackberry Jam

Directions

Use Raspberry Sugar Free jam instead of the Blackberry listed in the ingredients. Strawberry is great too!

1. Preheat oven to 325°F. Prepare two cookie sheets with silpats or parchment paper.
2. In a small bowl combine the peanut butter, granular sugar substitute, egg, vanilla, baking soda and salt. Blend together with a fork until thoroughly combined, about 3 minutes.
3. Using a 2 tbsp scoop or measure, divide dough into 18 balls on two cookie sheets placing about 2 inches apart. Bake for 10 minutes, remove from oven and make an indentation with the back of a small spoon (a round teaspoon works great) then drop one teaspoon of sugar-free jam into the well. Put back in the oven for another 10 minutes. Cool on the pan for 15 minutes then place on a wire rack. Cookies will keep in an airtight container in the refriferator for 1 week.

Nutritional Information

- Protein : 3.5g
- Fat : 7.8g
- Fiber : 1.6g
- Calories :101

Pear Tart

Servings: 6 | Prep: 40 m | Style: Other | Cook: 30 m

Ingredients

- 3/4 cup Whole Grain Soy Flour
- 9 tbsps Sucralose Based Sweetener (Sugar Substitute)
- 4 tbsps Unsalted Butter Stick
- 11 oz Cream Cheese
- 1 tbsp Sour Cream (Cultured)
- 2 small (approx 3 per lb) Pear
- 1 fl oz (no ice) Brandy
- 1/2 tsp Pure Almond Extract
- 1/2 tsp Ginger (Ground)
- 2 tbsps Sugar Free Apricot Preserves
- 1 large Egg (Whole)
- 2 tsps Tap Water
- 1 oz Almonds

Directions

1. Preheat oven to 350°F.
2. For crust: In a food processor, pulse flour and 2 tablespoons sugar substitute to combine, about 10 seconds. Add butter and pulse until mixture resembles a coarse meal, about 30 seconds.
3. Add 3 ounces cream cheese and the sour cream and pulse until the dough starts to come together, about 30 more seconds. Put dough on the bottom and up the sides of an ungreased 10 tart pan.
4. Prick dough about 15 times with a fork and chill in freezer while preparing filling.
5. For filling: In a small bowl, toss pear slices with 1 tablespoon of the sugar substitute, Cognac, 1/4 teaspoon of the almond extract and ginger until evenly distributed. Set aside.

67

6. In a large bowl with an electric mixer on high speed, beat 8 ounces cream cheese at room temperature and 1/3 cup sugar substitute until soft and creamy, about 3 minutes. Add egg and remaining 1/4 teaspoon almond extract; beat until smooth, 1 minute more (scrape down sides of bowl as necessary).
7. Pour cream cheese mixture into chilled tart shell. Arrange pears on top of cream cheese mixture in slightly overlapping concentric circles. If there is liquid left from the pears, pour it evenly over the tart.
8. Bake for 30 minutes, or until cheese mixture is just set. Remove from oven and place on a wire rack to cool.
9. Melt jam with water over medium heat. Brush over hot tart and sprinkle with almonds. Let tart cool completely before serving.

Nutritional Information

- Protein : 8.5g
- Fat : 30g
- Fiber : 2.8g
- Calories :373

Peppermint-Chocolate Truffles

Servings: 6 | Prep: 20 m | Style: American

Ingredients

- 4 oz Sugar Free Chocolate Chips
- 2 tbsps Heavy Cream
- 1 tbsp Unsalted Butter Stick
- 10 Bob's Starlight Mints Peppermint Sugar Free Candy
- 1 tbsp Vanilla Extract

Directions

1. Sugar-free striped hard peppermint candies can be found at some grocery stores or at specialty candy stores. Unwrap them and place them in a plastic bag then crush with a rolling pin or hammer before using.
2. Place chocolate in a small microwavable bowl; set aside. Place cream and butter in another small microwavable bowl; set aside.
3. Microwave chocolate for 30 seconds on medium; repeat for another 30 seconds. Microwave the bowl of chocolate a third time, along with the bowl of cream and butter, for another 30 seconds. Remove and pour the hot cream and butter mixture over the partially melted chocolate; let sit 1 minute. Stir to completely melt the chocolate and smooth the mixture. Add extract and thoroughly mix. If the chocolate isn't completely melted, return to the microwave for an additional 20 seconds.
4. Place the bowl in the refrigerator, covered with plastic wrap, for about 1 hour or until firm.
5. Working quickly to avoid melting, form 12 equal-size balls of the chocolate mixture with your fingers, immediately roll in a small amount of unsweetened cocoa powder or roll each in the peppermint candies (optional) to coat evenly. Set on a serving plate. Serve right away or refrigerate in an airtight container for up to 5 days. 2 truffles per serving.

Nutritional Information

- Protein : 1.1g
- Fat : 9.9g
- Fiber : 1.9g
- Calories :116

Pineapple-Coconut Granita

Servings: 4 | Prep: 105 m | Style: Other | Cook: 5 m

Ingredients

- 1/2 fruit Pineapple
- 1/2 cup Sucralose Based Sweetener (Sugar Substitute)
- 1/2 cup Tap Water
- 3/4 tsp Coconut Extract

Directions

1. In a food processor, pulse the pineapple until very smooth, about 2 minutes.
2. In a small saucepan over high heat, dissolve sugar substitute in water. Remove from heat. Add pineapple purée and coconut extract, stirring to combine. Pour the mixture into a 9 x13 pan.
3. Place the pan in freezer for 30 minutes or until ice crystals begin to form. Using a fork, break up ice and return to freezer. Continue breaking up ice crystals every 30 minutes until mixture is granular and completely frozen, about 1 1/2 hours.
4. Once the mixture is frozen cover the pan with plastic wrap, or if making a day ahead, place granita in a plastic storage container with a lid and store in freezer.
5. To serve, remove granita from freezer and allow to thaw for 2-3 minutes, breaking up any large ice crystals.

Nutritional Information

- Protein : 0.6g
- Fat : 0.1g
- Fiber : 1.6g
- Calories :71

Pineapple-Mango Layer Cake

Servings: 8 | Prep: 50 m | Style: American | Cook: 20 m

Ingredients

- 1/2 fruit Pineapple
- 1/2 cup sliced Mangos
- 1 cup Whole Grain Soy Flour
- 1 tsp Baking Powder (Straight Phosphate, Double Acting)
- 1/4 tsp Salt
- 6 large Eggs (Whole)
- 3/4 cup Sucralose Based Sweetener (Sugar Substitute)
- 2 tsps Pure Almond Extract
- 1/4 cup Unsalted Butter Stick
- 1/2 cup Heavy Cream
- 1 tbsp Sucralose Based Sweetener (Sugar Substitute)

Directions

1. For cake: Preheat oven to 350°F. Line two 8-inch-round cake pans with parchment paper, grease and dust with soy flour. Core the pineapple (cut off green outsides) and peel the mango. Dice all or leave about half of the pineapple in half-rings and half of the mango in slices for a decorative top; set aside.
2. In a medium bowl, whisk together soy flour, baking powder and salt. Separate the egg yolks from the whites. Set yolks aside. In a large bowl with an electric mixer on medium speed, beat whites until frothy, about 3 minutes. Slowly add 3/4 cup (12 Tbsp) sugar substitute and continue beating until stiff, but not dry, peaks form, about 4 minutes.
3. In a small bowl, whisk together yolks, almond extract and melted butter. Slowly pour yolk mixture into the beaten egg whites and continue mixing on medium speed until yolks are combined, about 1 minute. In three additions, gently fold the

71

dry ingredients into the egg white mixture using a rubber spatula. Divide batter in prepared pans; smooth tops.

4. Bake until a toothpick inserted in centers comes out clean, about 20 minutes. Cool on wire rack for 5 minutes, then turn out to cool completely.

5. To assemble: In a small bowl with an electric mixer on medium, whip heavy cream with 1 tablespoon sugar substitute until soft peaks form, about 3 minutes. Place one cake layer on a serving plate. Spread half the whipped cream over cake and place diced pineapple and mango pieces all around. Place second layer over whipped cream. Top with remaining whipped cream and decorate top with pieces or sliced pineapple and mango.

6. For a decorative top: Starting at the edge of the cake, arrange fruit in concentric circles, alternating pineapple and mango slices. Cut into 8 servings.

Nutritional Information

- Protein : 9.2g
- Fat : 17.2g
- Fiber : 2.1g
- Calories :256

Pinwheel Cookies

Servings: 28 | Prep: 45 m | Style: Other | Cook: 18 m

Ingredients

- 4 oz Cream Cheese
- 2 tbsps Unsalted Butter Stick
- 2 tbsps Sour Cream (Cultured)
- 4 tsps Sucralose Based Sweetener (Sugar Substitute)
- 1 cup Whole Grain Soy Flour
- 1 tsp Baking Powder (Straight Phosphate, Double Acting)

- 1/4 cup chopped English Walnuts
- 2 oz Sugar Free Chocolate Chips
- 1/4 tsp Cinnamon

Directions

1. Line two baking sheets with aluminum foil; set aside.
2. In a bowl, with an electric mixer on low, mix cream cheese, butter, sour cream and sugar substitute until smooth, about 4 minutes. With the mixer still on low, sift flour and baking powder together and gradually add until dough pulls away from the side. Form dough into a rectangle, cover with plastic wrap and refrigerate for 20 minutes.
3. While dough is chilling, combine walnuts, chocolate chips and cinnamon. Roll dough between two pieces of plastic wrap to a rectangle measuring 8 x11.
4. Before removing the dough from the freezer, preheat oven to 350°F. Remove top layer of plastic wrap. Sprinkle chocolate-nut filling evenly over dough, leaving a 1/2-inch border along the longer side.
5. Roll dough up jelly roll style, beginning with the long side and using bottom sheet of plastic wrap to help roll the dough into a cylinder. Place in freezer and chill for 10 minutes.
6. Using a sharp knife, cut roll into 1/2-inch slices. Arrange slices on prepared baking sheets. Bake 18 minutes, or until lightly golden and set.

Nutritional Information

- Protein : 1.5g
- Fat : 4.2g
- Fiber : 0.5g
- Calories :50

Pistachio Butter Cookies

Servings: 24 | Prep: 20 m | Style: American | Cook: 16 m

Ingredients

- 1/2 cup Dry Roasted Pistachio Nuts (Without Salt Added)
- 1/4 cup, dry, yield Oatmeal
- 1/3 cup Sucralose Based Sweetener (Sugar Substitute)
- 1/3 cup Whole Grain Wheat Flour
- 1/3 cup Whole Grain Soy Flour
- 1/8 tsp Salt
- 1/4 tsp Baking Powder (Straight Phosphate, Double Acting)
- 1/2 cup Unsalted Butter Stick
- 1 large Egg (Whole)
- 1 tsp Vanilla Extract
- 1/3 second spray Original Canola Cooking Spray

Directions

1. Preheat oven to 375°F. Lightly grease a baking sheet with oil spray.
2. Process pistachios, oatmeal, sugar substitute, flours, salt and baking powder in a food processor until nuts and oatmeal are finely ground, about 1 minute. Add butter, egg and vanilla processing until combined, about 15 seconds, scraping down sides if necessary. Chill dough for 15 minutes, until firm.
3. Roll dough into 24 balls and place on prepared sheet. Flatten with palm of hand to about 1/8 thick. Bake cookies until bottoms and edges are deep golden, 14-16 minutes. Cool cookies on baking sheet 1 minute before transferring to wire racks to cool completely. Store in an airtight container.

Nutritional Information

- Protein : 1.5g

- Fat : 5.5g
- Fiber : 0.6g
- Calories :66

Pumpkin Cheesecake

Servings: 10 | Prep: 240 m | Style: American | Cook: 45 m

Ingredients

- 24 oz Cream Cheese
- 15 oz Pumpkin (Without Salt, Canned)
- 2/3 cup Sucralose Based Sweetener (Sugar Substitute)
- 1/2 tsp Vanilla Extract
- 1/2 tsp Cinnamon
- 1/4 tsp Ginger (Ground)
- 3 large Eggs (Whole)

Directions

1. Be sure to use pure pumpkin purée, not pumpkin pie mix, which is sweetened with sugar.
2. Heat oven to 325°F. Spray an 8x3-inch deep cake pan with vegetable cooking spray. Line bottom with a round of parchment or wax paper; spray paper; set aside.
3. In a large bowl, with an electric mixer on medium, beat cream cheese until smooth. Add pumpkin purée, sugar substitute, vanilla, cinnamon and ginger; beat until smooth.
4. Beat in eggs one at a time, just until combined. Pour batter into prepared pan. Place cake pan in a deep roasting pan and carefully pour in enough boiling water into roasting pan to reach halfway up sides of cake pan. Bake 42-45 minutes, until cake is just set in center. Turn off oven, open door and let stand in oven 15 minutes. Remove cake pan from water

bath and transfer to a wire rack; cool completely. Run a knife around edge of cake, cover and refrigerate until chilled (4 hours or overnight).

5. To remove cake from pan, dip bottom of pan into hot water for just a few seconds to loosen. Place serving platter over top and invert. Remove pan and peel off paper. Garnish with mint and pecans, if desired.

Nutritional Information

- Protein : 6.4g
- Fat : 24.9g
- Fiber : 1.3g
- Calories :276

Pumpkin Mousse

Servings: 8 | Prep: 25 m | Style: American

Ingredients

- 1 package (1 oz) Gelatin Powder (Unsweetened)
- 1/4 cup Tap Water
- 2 tsps Pumpkin Pie Spice
- 15 oz Pumpkin (Without Salt, Canned)
- 1 1/2 cups Heavy Cream
- 1/2 cup Sucralose Based Sweetener (Sugar Substitute)
- 2 tsps Vanilla Extract

Directions

1. In small bowl, sprinkle gelatin over cool water, let sit 5 minutes until gelatin softens. Meanwhile, in a small skillet over medium heat, toast pumpkin pie spice 1 2 minutes until fragrant, stirring frequently. Reduce heat to low, stir in

gelatin mixture and cook 1-2 minutes more until gelatin melts. Remove from heat; cool to room temperature.
2. Place pumpkin purée in a large bowl.
3. In another large bowl, with an electric mixer on high, beat cream, sugar substitute and vanilla until soft peaks form. With a rubber spatula, slowly fold in cooled gelatin mixture.
4. In three additions, gently fold whipped cream mixture into pumpkin purée.
5. Divide mousse into 8 dessert glasses. Chill 2 hours.

Nutritional Information

- Protein: 2.3g
- Fat: 16.8g
- Fiber: 1.5g
- Calories: 185

Pumpkin Pie Topped with Meringue and Toasted Nuts

Servings: 8 | Prep: 15 m | Style: American | Cook: 60 m

Ingredients

- 1/3 cup 100% Stone Ground Whole Wheat Pastry Flour
- 1/2 cup chopped Pecan Nuts
- 1 cup Sucralose Based Sweetener (Sugar Substitute)
- 6 tbsps Unsalted Butter Stick
- 1 fl oz Tap Water
- 15 oz Pumpkin (Without Salt, Canned)
- 1 tsp Cinnamon
- 3/4 tsp Ginger (Ground)
- 1/4 tsp Cloves (Ground)
- 1/4 tsp Salt

- 2 large Eggs (Whole)
- 1 1/4 cups Heavy Cream
- 3 large Egg Whites
- 1/4 tsp Cream Of Tartar
- 1/4 cup Sucralose Based Sweetener (Sugar Substitute)
- 1/2 cup chopped Pecan Nuts
- 2 servings All Purpose Low-Carb Baking Mix

Directions

Use the Atkins recipe to make All Purpose Low-Carb Baking Mix for this recipe. 1 serving =1/3 cup so you will need 2/3 cup

For pie:

1. Heat oven to 425ºF.
2. In a large bowl whisk together flour, 2/3 cup baking mix, pecans (chop finely) and 1/4 cup sugar substitute. Cut in butter with a pastry blender or two knives until butter pieces are about the size of peas. Add the ice water; stir to combine.
3. Transfer crust mixture to a 9-inch pie plate. Press along bottom and sides of pie plate to form a crust. Place in freezer to harden, about 15 minutes.
4. Cover crust with aluminum foil and bake 15 minutes; remove from oven and take off foil. Reduce oven to 375ºF.
5. In a bowl, whisk pumpkin purée, 3/4 cup sugar substitute, ground cinnamon, ginger, cloves, and salt to combine. Mix in eggs, one at a time. Add heavy cream and mix well.
6. Pour filling into partially baked pie crust. Cover crust edge with aluminum foil. Bake 40 minutes, or until filling is set but still a little jiggly in the middle. Cool on a wire rack while you make the meringue but turn the oven down to 350°F.

For meringue and toasted nut topping:

1. Whip egg whites and cream of tartar with an electric beater until frothy. Slowly add 1/4 cup granulated sugar substitute until fully incorporated then whip at high speed until stiff glossy peaks form. Top pie with meringue and then sprinkle the 1/2 cup finely chopped nuts on top. Place in the oven and continue to bake for 15-20 minutes until the nuts are toasted and browned.
2. Cool on a wire rack until ready to serve. The pie may be made up to 3 days prior to serving, but do not add the meringue until you are ready to serve. Be sure the pie has warmed to room temperature if previously chilled before adding and cooking the meringue and nuts (otherwise your pie plate may crack with the sudden change in temperature). The meringue topping will not keep more than a day once made.

Nutritional Information

- Protein: 13.9g
- Fat: 34.8g
- Fiber: 4.5g
- Calories: 423

Pumpkin Pie with Pecan Crust

Servings: 8 | Prep: 15 m | Style: American | Cook: 44 m

Ingredients

- 1/3 cup 100% Stone Ground Whole Wheat Pastry Flour
- 1/2 cup chopped Pecan Nuts
- 1 cup Sucralose Based Sweetener (Sugar Substitute)
- 6 tbsps Unsalted Butter Stick
- 1 fl oz Tap Water
- 15 oz Pumpkin (Without Salt, Canned)

- 1 tsp Cinnamon
- 3/4 tsp Ginger (Ground)
- 1/4 tsp Cloves (Ground)
- 1/4 tsp Salt
- 2 large Eggs (Whole)
- 1 1/4 cups Heavy Cream
- 2 servings All Purpose Low-Carb Baking Mix

Directions

Use the Atkins recipe to make All Purpose Low-Carb Baking Mix for this recipe. 1 serving =1/3 cup so you will need 2/3 cup.

1. Heat oven to 425ºF.
2. In a large bowl whisk together flour, 2/3 cup baking mix, pecans (chop finely) and 1/4 cup sugar substitute. Cut in butter with a pastry blender or two knives until butter pieces are about the size of peas. Add the ice water; stir to combine.
3. Transfer crust mixture to a 9-inch pie plate. Press along bottom and sides of pie plate to form a crust. Place in freezer to harden, about 15 minutes.
4. Cover crust with aluminum foil and bake 15 minutes; remove from oven and take off foil. Reduce oven to 375ºF.
5. In a bowl, whisk pumpkin purée, 3/4 cup sugar substitute, ground cinnamon, ginger, cloves, and salt to combine. Mix in eggs, one at a time. Add heavy cream and mix well.
6. Pour filling into partially baked pie crust. Cover crust edge with aluminum foil. Bake 40 minutes, or until filling is set but still a little jiggly in the middle. Cook on a wire rack. Makes 8 servings.

Nutritional Information

- Protein: 11.9g
- Fat: 29.4g
- Fiber: 3.8g

- Calories: 364

Pumpkin Pots

Servings: 6 | Prep: 10 m | Style: American | Cook: 38 m

Ingredients

- 2 large Eggs (Whole)
- 2 large Egg Yolks
- 1 14 oz can Coconut Cream
- 1 tsp Vanilla Extract
- 15 oz Pumpkin (Without Salt, Canned)
- 1/4 cup Xylitol
- 1 pinch Stevia
- 1/4 cup Sugar Free Maple Flavored Syrup
- 1 tsp Ginger (Ground)
- 1 tsp Cinnamon
- 1/4 tsp Nutmeg (Ground)
- 3/4 tsp Salt

Directions

1. For this recipe, add or delete spices as desired (the combination given is generally a pumpkin pie spice mixture). Add the stevia sparingly, taste the recipe before baking if you are unsure and add more stevia or sugar-free maple syrup if more sweetness or maple flavor is desired; whisk in any additional thoroughly. Additionally, this recipe can easily be made by substituting heavy cream for the coconut milk; add 1.3g NC per serving.
2. Preheat oven to 400°F. Lightly grease 6 ramekins; set aside. You will also need a pan big enough to accommodate all the ramekins and deep enough to hold 1-inch of water without spilling into the ramekins.

3. Whisk the whole eggs and yolks with the coconut milk and vanilla in a medium bowl. Set aside.
4. In a medium sauce pot combine the pumpkin, granular sugar substitutes, maple syrup, ginger, ground cinnamon, nutmeg and salt. Cook over medium-high heat until reduced slightly, fragrant and shiny; about 15 minutes stirring often to prevent burning on the bottom of the pan. Remove from heat and quickly whisk in the egg mixture.
5. Divide mixture into 6 ramekins (do not overfill) and place in a deep sided pan. Fill the pan with hot water until it reaches about 1-inch up the side of the ramekins. Place in oven and bake for 10 minutes at 400°F then reduce heat to 300°F and cook an additional 25-30 minutes or until the centers jiggle only slightly in the center. Remove from oven and allow to sit in the water bath to cool to room temperature. These are wonderful eaten warm about 20 minutes after baking or cold after being refrigerated for at least 3 hours or up to 2 days. Store leftovers in the refrigerator covered with plastic wrap and eat within 1 week. Top with a dollop of whipped cream just before serving if desired.

Nutritional Information

- Protein: 4.5g
- Fat: 8.6g
- Fiber: 10.4g
- Calories: 147

Pumpkin-Spice Brownies

Servings: 16 | Prep: 10 m | Style: American | Cook: 30 m

Ingredients

- 2 oz Unsweetened Baking Chocolate Squares
- 1/2 cup Unsalted Butter Stick
- 1 tbsp Cocoa Powder (Unsweetened)
- 24 tsps Erythritol
- 2 tsps Vanilla Extract
- 4 large Eggs (Whole)
- 4 tbsps Organic High Fiber Coconut Flour
- 1/4 tsp Baking Soda
- 1/4 tsp Salt
- 1/2 tsp Cinnamon
- 8 oz Cream Cheese
- 1/3 cup Sucralose Based Sweetener (Sugar Substitute)
- 2/3 cup Pumpkin (Without Salt, Canned)
- 1 1/2 tsps Pumpkin Pie Spice

Directions

You will need 4 oz or 1/2 cup erythritol for this recipe. Powdered pure erythritol may be purchased from specialty stores or online. Granulated erythritol is more easily found in health food stores and may also easily be powdered by placing it in a blender and pulsing for 5 seconds. Be sure to use powdered erythritol and measure after it is powdered. 4oz = 1 cup powdered erythritol. Sucralose may be used for the brownie (use 1 full cup) and add 1.5g NC to each serving total; some people find the combination of chocolate and sucralose to be bitter.

1. Preheat an oven to 350°F. Grease an 8x8-inch pan.
2. Melt the butter and chocolate in a small bowl at 30 second intervals in the microwave until melted. Thoroughly blend the chocolate and butter together then add in the cocoa powder and powdered erythritol (1 cup made from 1/2 cup granulated) and continue to blend until smooth. Add 1 teaspoon vanilla and 3 eggs; whisk until incorporated. Combine the coconut flour, baking soda, salt

and cinnamon in a small bowl. Add to the chocolate mixture and stir until thickened. Set the brownie mixture aside.

3. Using a hand blender cream the cream cheese with the sucralose in a small bowl. Add 1 egg, pumpkin purée, pumpkin spice blend and 1 teaspoon vanilla; beat until smooth.
4. Spread 2/3 of the brownie mixture into the prepared pan. Then pour the cream cheese mixture over the top. Drop the remaining 1/3 of the brownie batter by spoonfuls over the cream cheese mixture and then take a knife and gently swirl the layers together. Bake for 30 minutes until a tooth pick inserted in the center comes out clean. Allow to cool before cutting. Best served at room temperature but keep refrigerated in an airtight container for up to 1 week.

Nutritional Information

- Protein: 3.4g
- Fat: 14g
- Fiber: 1.7g
- Calories: 150

Raspberry Parfait

Servings: 2 | Prep: 5 m | Style: American

Ingredients

- 1/2 cup Heavy Cream
- 4 oz Mascarpone
- 2 individual packets Sucralose Based Sweetener (Sugar Substitute)
- 1/2 cup Raspberries

Directions

1. Beat 1/2 cup heavy crem until soft peaks form.
2. Add 4 oz mascarpone and 2 pakcets of sweetener. Beat just until smooth.
3. Using 1/2 cup raspberries, layer with the dairy mixture in 2 parfait glasses.

Nutritional Information

- Protein: 5.6g
- Fat: 48.7g
- Fiber: 2g
- Calories: 470

Root Beer Float

Servings: 1 | Prep: 5 m | Style: American

Ingredients

- 1 can Diet Root Beer
- 2 tbsps Heavy Cream

Directions

1. Combine half of the root beer can with 7 ice cubes and cream in a blender. Purée until smooth.
2. Add the remaining root beer can; pulse to incorporate. Enjoy!

Nutritional Information

- Protein: 0.6g
- Fat: 11.1g
- Fiber: 0g
- Calories: 104

Snickerdoodle Cupcakes

Servings: 8 | Prep: 25 m | Style: American | Cook: 22 m

Ingredients

- 3/4 cup Unsalted Butter Stick
- 1/4 cup Sucralose Based Sweetener (Sugar Substitute)
- 2 large Eggs (Whole)
- 2 tsps Vanilla Extract
- 3 tbsps Heavy Cream
- 1 fl oz Tap Water
- 4 tbsps Organic High Fiber Coconut Flour
- 3/4 cup Almond Meal Flour
- 3/4 tsp Baking Powder (Straight Phosphate, Double Acting)
- 1/8 tsp Salt
- 2 tsps Cinnamon
- 2 large Egg Whites
- 1/3 cup Xylitol

Directions

This recipe is suitable for all phases except for the first two weeks of Induction due to the nuts. This recipe uses xylitol for the frosting. Be sure to measure it first and then powder it in a blender before use.

Cupcakes:

1. Preheat oven to 350°F. Prepare a muffin tin with 8 foil or paper liners. Beat 1/4 cup softened butter and sucralose until light and fluffy. Add 2 whole eggs, 1 tsp vanilla, heavy cream, 2 Tbsp water and coconut flour.

2. In a separate bowl whisk to combine the almond flour, baking powder, salt and 2 tsp cinnamon. Combine the almond mixture with the egg mixture and blend until smooth. Fill the muffin wells and bake for 20-25 minutes until cooked through. Allow to sit in the muffin tin for 5 minutes then remove to a baking rack to cool. Frost once cooled.

Buttercream Frosting:

1. Prepare a pan with simmering water fitted with another pan over the top (Bain Marie). Do not allow the surface of the water to touch the bottom of the top pan. To the top pan (a metal mixing bowl works great for this purpose) add 2 egg whites (be sure there are no yolks), a dash of cream of tartar, 1 tsp water and 1/3 cup xylitol (it is not necessary to powder it). Whisk this mixture continuously for 5-10 minutes over the water bath until all the xylitol has dissolved.
2. Pour this mixture into a separate bowl and whip with a blender until stiff fluffy peaks form. Add 1 tsp vanilla, blend to incorporate. The frosting may be used, as is, immediately (it does not store well) as a marshmallow frosting - dust the cupcakes with cinnamon as a garnish.

For butter cream:

1. To the marshmallow frosting, continue to beat on medium speed, begin adding about 1/2 cup butter 1 tablespoon at a time (allow to beat for 1 minute between each addition of butter). The frosting may break down and get soupy looking, continue to add butter and beat until it comes together (more butter may be necessary, 1 tablespoon at a time).
2. Add 1-2 tsp cinnamon (to taste, optional) and blend to combine. Buttercream should be used immediately by piping onto the cooled cupcake with a pastry bag and fancy tip or by simply cutting the corner of a plastic

87

bag. Buttercream frosted cupcakes may be refrigerated in an airtight container for up to 5 days. Serve at room temperature dusted with cinnamon.

Nutritional Information

- Protein: 5.5g
- Fat: 26.3g
- Fiber: 10.7g
- Calories: 297

Spiced Coconut Bark

Servings: 12 | Prep: 15 m | Style: American |

Ingredients

- 7 oz Sugar Free Chocolate Chips
- 1 tsp Cinnamon
- 1/8 tsp Chili Powder
- 1/4 tsp Coarse Kosher Salt
- 5 tbsps Dried Coconut

Directions

1. Melt chocolate in the microwave at 30 second intervals (about 3 times) until it begins to melt. Stir in between and do not over heat.
2. Stir in ground cinnamon and chipotle pepper (as deisred for taste, amounts given are delicious but feel free to play with different levels to your taste). Stir in 2 tablespoons shredded coconut. Pour onto parchment paper, spread out evenly into a 6x8-inch rectangle and sprinkle remaining 3 tablespoons shredded coconut on top. Sprinkle coarse Kosher salt on top as well (optional).

3. Place in the refrigerator for 10-15 minutes to firm up then divide into 12 equal portions (squares of 2x2 inches are best for portioning).

Nutritional Information

- Protein: 0.6g
- Fat: 6.9g
- Fiber: 1.6g
- Calories: 83

Spiced Snack Cake

Servings: 9 | Prep: 25 m | Style: Other | Cook: 25 m

Ingredients

- 1 tsp rounded Coffee (Instant Powder, Decaffeinated)
- 1/4 cup Tap Water
- 4 tbsps Heavy Cream
- 1 cup Whole Grain Soy Flour
- 2 tsps Cinnamon
- 1/4 tsp Cloves (Ground)
- 1 1/2 tsps Baking Powder (Straight Phosphate, Double Acting)
- 1 tsp Cocoa Powder (Unsweetened)
- 1 tbsp Ginger (Ground)
- 1/2 tsp Allspice Ground
- 1/4 tsp Salt
- 2 large Eggs (Whole)
- 1/2 cup Unsalted Butter Stick
- 2 tsps Vanilla Extract
- 1/2 cup Sucralose Based Sweetener (Sugar Substitute)

Directions

1. Heat oven to 350°F. Lightly butter an 8-inch square baking pan and line bottom with parchment paper; set aside.
2. Combine coffee and hot water in a cup; stir until coffee is dissolved. Cool. Stir in cream; set aside.
3. In a medium bowl, combine soy flour, ginger, cinnamon, baking powder, cocoa powder, allspice, cloves and salt; set aside.
4. In a large bowl, with electric mixer on low, beat butter just until creamy. Increase speed to medium-high and beat butter until smooth and light in color, 1 1/2 to 2 minutes.
5. Gradually beat in sugar substitute. Add eggs one at a time, beating well after each addition and scraping sides of bowl as necessary. Beat in vanilla. Reduce speed to medium-low.
6. Add dry mixture in three additions, alternating with the coffee-cream mixture and beginning and ending with dry mix. Beat just until combined. Scrape down sides of bowl and beat 10 seconds more.
7. Spoon batter into prepared pan and smooth top. Bake until a toothpick inserted in center of cake comes out clean, about 25 minutes. Cool on a wire rack. Run a knife around edge of pan, and invert onto wire rack; peel off parchment paper.
8. Invert again onto a cutting board. Using a serrated knife, cut into 9 squares. Dust with cinnamon, and serve warm or at room temperature.

Nutritional Information

- Protein: 5g
- Fat: 15.7g
- Fiber: 1.4g
- Calories: 183

Star Spangled Berry Trifle

Servings: 12 | Prep: 180 m | Style: American

Ingredients

- 1 fl oz Fresh Lemon Juice
- 1 fl oz Tap Water
- 2 1/2 tsps Vanilla Extract
- 1 tsp Pure Almond Extract
- 9 tbsps Xylitol
- 2 pinches Stevia
- 1/2 cup Organic High Fiber Coconut Flour
- 1/2 tsp Salt
- 2 large Eggs (Whole)
- 2 cups Heavy Cream
- 1 cup Coconut Milk Unsweetened
- 12 large Egg Whites
- 1 tsp Thick-It-Up
- 3 cup sliceds Strawberries
- 3 cups Blackberries

Directions

1. Preheat oven to 350°F. Prepare a large sheet pan with with parchment paper. Set aside.
2. Beat egg whites until frothy. Add the lemon juice and water. Continue to beat and slowly add in 4 tablespoons xylitol, a pinch of stevia, and 1 teaspoon each of vanilla and almond extracts. Fold in the coconut flour and salt until just incorporated. Place mixture on top of the parchment and smooth out with a spatula, making sure it stays on the parchment.. Bake for 15-20 minutes, remove and allow to cool 5 minutes on the pan. Quickly turn the cake over and gently lift the parchment off of the cake, set the cake aside to cool.
3. While the cake is baking make pastry cream. Place 1 cup heavy cream and 1 cup coconut milk into a 1 quart pan. Add 2 tablespoons xylitol and a pinch of stevia along with a pinch

of salt. Heat over medium high heat until bubbles just start to appear around the edges of the pan.

4. In a small bowl combine the eggs, Thick-It-Up and 2 tablespoons xylitol. Whisk to combine. Continue whisking and slowly add about half of the hot cream mixture to the eggs. Return egg mixture to the rest of the cream in the pan. Cook for 5-10 minutes until the mixture has boiled for about 1-2 minutes and thickened; stir continuously. Strain through a mesh strainer into a bowl , place plastic wrap on the surface and set aside. Allow to cool to room temperature (speed this up by placing over an ice water bath); about 30 minutes, add in 1 teaspoon vanilla extract, and place into the refrigerator to cool for at least 2 hours.

5. Whip the cream with 1 tablespoon xylitol and 1/2 teaspoon vanilla until fully whipped. Fold whipped cream into cold pastry cream. Additional stevia may be added to taste.

6. Assemble Trifle. Cut out stars or other designs from the cake; set aside. Cut up the remaining pieces and gently mix into the pastry cream. Start by layering the strawberries on the bottom. Add 1/2 of the pastry cream mixture then place the blackberries on top of the pastry cream. Top it off with a final layer of pastry cream and decorate top with the reserved cake stars. If desired, place a few reserved stars along the inside of the bowl as you layer the ingredients up. The serving size is about 1 cup.

Nutritional Information

- Protein: 6.9g
- Fat: 17g
- Fiber: 13.6g
- Calories: 247

Strawberries and Cream Cupcakes

Servings: 10 | Prep: 10 m | Style: American | Cook: 20 m

Ingredients

- 7 oz Unsalted Butter Stick
- 1/4 cup Xylitol
- 3 large Eggs (Whole)
- 1 tsp Vanilla Extract
- 1/3 cup Organic High Fiber Coconut Flour
- 1/4 cup Heavy Cream
- 1 1/2 fl ozs Tap Water
- 1 cup Almond Meal Flour
- 1 tsp Baking Powder (Straight Phosphate, Double Acting)
- 1/4 tsp Salt
- 8 oz Cream Cheese
- 1/2 cup Sucralose Based Sweetener (Sugar Substitute)
- 2 tbsps Sugar Free Strawberry Jam
- 10 small (1" dia) Strawberries

Directions

Xylitol usually comes in granular form. Please measure first and then powder in a blender before using in this recipe. You may substitute granular sucralose 1:1 for the xylitol in the cupcakes but please add 0.6g NC per serving to the total g NC.

Cupcakes:

1. Preheat oven to 350°F. Line a muffin tin with 10 paper or foil liners. Beat 1/3 cup (about 3oz) softened butter and the powdered xylitol until light and fluffy, about 3 minutes. Add one egg at a time until incorporated, then the vanilla.

2. Add the coconut flour and blend until incorporated. Add the heavy cream and water and continue to blend until smooth.
3. Combine the almond flour, baking powder and 1/4 tsp salt. Add to the egg mixture forming a thickened batter.
4. Divide equally into the 10 muffin liners and bake for 20-25 minutes until golden brown on top and baked through. Allow to cool.

Frosting:

1. Beat 1/2 cup (about 4 oz) butter, cream cheese and a dash of salt for about 2 minutes. Add the sucralose and 2 tablespoons sugar-free strawberry jam. 2-3 drops of red food coloring may be added for a pinker color.
2. Using a piping bag and fancy tip or simply a quart-sized plastic bag with a corner cut off, pipe the frosting onto the cupcakes and garnish with a strawberry.
3. The cupcakes can be kept in an airtight container refrigerated for up to one week. Serve at room temperature.

Nutritional Information

- Protein: 6.5g
- Fat: 33.7g
- Fiber: 7.5g
- Calories: 364

Strawberries with French Cream

Servings: 4 | Prep: 10 m | Style: French

Ingredients

- 1/2 cup Heavy Cream
- 1 tbsp Sucralose Based Sweetener (Sugar Substitute)
- 3 tbsps Sour Cream (Cultured)
- 4 pint as purchased, yields Strawberries

Directions

1. With an electric mixer on high speed, beat cream and sugar substitute until soft peaks form, about 4 minutes.
2. Beat in sour cream until well-mixed. Serve with berries.

Nutritional Information

- Protein: 1.6g
- Fat: 1.6g
- Fiber: 2.3g
- Calories: 159

Strawberry Granita

Servings: 6 | Prep: 120 m | Style: Italian

Ingredients

- 16 oz Strawberries
- 1 cup Tap Water
- 3/4 cup Sucralose Based Sweetener (Sugar Substitute)
- 1 tbsp Fresh Lemon Juice

Directions

1. In a food processor fitted with a steel blade, purée the strawberries. Add water, sugar substitute and lemon juice. Pulse to combine.
2. Pour mixture into a 9 by 13-inch baking pan. Place in freezer. Freeze 30 minutes.
3. Stir with fork. Freeze an additional 1 1/2 to 2 hours, scraping with a fork every 30 minutes (mixture should be granular) and breaking up any large pieces.

4. Serve in dessert bowls and garnish with mint sprigs, if desired.

Nutritional Information

- Protein: 0.5g
- Fat: 0.2g
- Fiber: 1.5g
- Calories: 37

Strawberry Shortcake Trifle

Servings: 12 | Prep: 100 m | Style: American | Cook: 20 m

Ingredients

- 1 1/2 cups Almond Meal Flour
- 1 tsp Baking Powder (Straight Phosphate, Double Acting)
- 4 tbsps Sucralose Based Sweetener (Sugar Substitute)
- 3 tbsps Unsalted Butter Stick
- 2 large Eggs (Whole)
- 2 cups Heavy Cream
- 1 individual packet Sucralose Based Sweetener (Sugar Substitute)
- 4 tsps Vanilla Extract
- 8 oz Cream Cheese
- 4 tbsps Sugar Free Apricot Preserves
- 2 cup sliceds Strawberries
- 1 oz Almonds

Directions

1. Preheat oven to 350°F. Spray a sheet pan with non-stick spray and set aside.

2. In a food processor, pulse the almond flour, baking powder and 2 teaspoons sugar substitute until mixed. Add the cold butter and pulse until it becomes crumbly. Add the eggs and 3 tablespoons of cream and pulse until the mixture is thoroughly combined, about 30 seconds.
3. Drop about 2 tablespoons mixture onto the sheet pan making 12 rounded biscuits. Bake for 20 minutes until tops crack and are golden on the edges. Allow to cool.
4. In a medium bowl beat the remaining cream, 2 tablespoons sugar substitute and 2 teaspoons vanilla extract until soft peaks form, about 3 to 4 minutes. Place one-third of the whipped cream in a small bowl and set aside.
5. Whisk 2 tablespoons sugar substitute and 2 teaspoons vanilla extract into cream cheese. With a rubber spatula, gently fold cream cheese into the remaining two-thirds of the whipped cream until well combined. Set aside.
6. Cut biscuits in half. Spread each with about 1 teaspoon jam, then cut into 1-inch pieces.

To assemble:

1. Spread one-third of the biscuit pieces on the bottom of a 2-quart glass dessert dish.
2. Spread half of the cream cheese mixture over biscuit pieces and top with 1 cup strawberries. Repeat.
3. Scatter remaining biscuit pieces over last layer of berries. Cover with reserved whipped cream. Top with remaining berries and scatter the toasted almonds on top. Chill for 1 hour for flavors to blend.

Nutritional Information

- Protein: 6.4g
- Fat: 32.5g
- Fiber: 2.2g
- Calories: 345

Strawberry-Rhubarb Pie

Servings: 8 | Prep: 135 m | Style: American | Cook: 15 m

Ingredients

- 4 stalks Rhubarb
- 1/2 cup Tap Water
- 1/3 cup Sucralose Based Sweetener (Sugar Substitute)
- 3 1/2 cup halves Strawberries
- 1/2 tsp Thick-It-Up
- 1/2 tsp Fresh Lemon Juice
- 1/8 tsp Salt
- 8 servings Atkins Cuisine Pie Crust

Directions

Use the Atkins recipe to make Atkins Cuisine Pie Crust for this recipe.

1. Prepare pie crust according to recipe. Pre-bake the pie shell.
2. Chop rhubarb into 1-inch pieces and place it in a medium saucepan over medium heat with the water and sugar substitute. Bring to a boil. Reduce the heat and simmer until rhubarb is very soft, about 10 to 15 minutes. Turn heat down to low.
3. Add berries, thickener, lemon juice and salt and stir until thickened, about 3 minutes. Pour filling into prepared pie shell.
4. Chill until set, about 2 hours. Serve with sweetened whipped cream, if desired. Makes 8 servings.

Nutritional Information

- Protein: 8.6g
- Fat: 13g
- Fiber: 3.4g

- Calories: 207

Sweet Potato-Pumpkin Purée

Servings: 12 | Prep: 20 m | Style: American | Cook: 65 m

Ingredients

- 3 large Egg Whites
- 5 tbsps Sucralose Based Sweetener (Sugar Substitute)
- 15 oz Pumpkin (Without Salt, Drained, Cooked, Boiled)
- 1/2 cup half Pecan Nuts
- 1 1/2 lbs Sweet Potato
- 1/2 cup Heavy Cream
- 1/2 tsp Salt
- 1/2 tsp Pumpkin Pie Spice
- 1/2 tsp Cinnamon
- 1/4 cup Unsalted Butter Stick

Directions

1. Heat oven to 250°F. Lightly butter a baking sheet.
2. Place egg whites in a medium mixing bowl; beat with an electric mixer at high speed until foamy. Gradually add sugar substitute and continue mixing just until soft peaks form. Spoon onto prepared baking sheet and spread with a spatula to ¼-inch thickness. Bake 35 minutes. Turn oven off; let meringue stand in oven for 45 minutes. Crush meringue and place in a bowl. Add pecans and toss gently to combine. Set aside.
3. While meringue is resting, place sweet potatoes in a medium saucepan. Cover with water to 2 inches above potatoes and bring to a boil. Cook until tender, about 20 minutes, and drain. Return saucepan to medium-high heat. Add potatoes,

butter, cream sugar substitute, salt, cinnamon, pumpkin pie spice and pumpkin puree. Stir to combine. Mash with a potato masher until smooth. Heat through, about 1 minute.

4. Transfer potato mixture to a serving dish and cover with meringue topping.

Nutritional Information

- Protein: 2.8g
- Fat: 10.7g
- Fiber: 3.2g
- Calories: 165

Tiramisu Cupcakes

Servings: 6 | Prep: 25 m | Style: Italian | Cook: 15 m

Ingredients

- 3 tbsps Unsalted Butter Stick
- 3 large Eggs (Whole)
- 1/4 cup Sucralose Based Sweetener (Sugar Substitute)
- 4 tsps Vanilla Extract
- 1 /4 cup Organic High Fiber Coconut Flour
- 1/4 tsp Baking Powder (Straight Phosphate, Double Acting)
- 1/4 tsp Salt
- 4 oz Mascarpone
- 5 tbsps Xylitol
- 1 1/4 tsp dries Coffee (Instant Powder)
- 1/2 cup Heavy Cream
- 1/2 fl oz Tap Water

Directions

Xylitol is used in combination with sucralose in this recipe to provide a more rounded sweetness. Xylitol usually comes granulated but is better incorporated if it is powdered before use. Please measure first then powder in a blender.

Cupcakes:

1. Preheat oven to 375°F. Prepare a muffin tin with paper or foil cups.
2. Using an electric mixer blend together the butter and sucralose until light and fluffy; about 2 minutes. Add eggs, 1 tsp vanilla, coconut flour, baking powder and salt. Blend until smooth then fill 6 muffin cups and bake for 15 minutes or until cooked through. Allow to sit for 5 minutes in the tin then place on a cooling rack.
3. Soaking syrup: combine 2 tsp vanilla, 2 Tbsp xylitol, 1 tsp espresso powder and 1 1/2 Tbsp water. Prick cupcakes with a tooth pick and pour 1 tsp soaking syrup per cupcake over the top.

Mascarpone Frosting:

1. Beat together the mascarpone cheese, 3 Tbsp xylitol, 1 tsp vanilla and 1/4 tsp espresso powder until smooth.
2. In a separate bowl whip the heavy creamy until stiff peaks form.
3. Fold the whipped cream into the mascarpone mixture until combined. Place mixture in a pastry bag fitted with a fancy tip or simply use a plastic sandwich bag with a corner cut off. Pipe the frosting onto the cooled cupcakes. Best if served the same day or they may be refrigerated overnight in an airtight container. Serve at room temperature dusted with cocoa powder and topped with crushed espresso beans if desired.

Nutritional Information

- Protein: 5.7g
- Fat: 25g

- Fiber: 11.7g
- Calories: 294

Tropical Raspberry Smoothie

Servings: 1 | Prep: 5 m | Style: Other

Ingredients

- 1/2 cup Coconut Cream
- 4 oz Firm Silken Tofu
- 1/2 cup Red Raspberries
- 2 tsps Sucralose Based Sweetener (Sugar Substitute)
- 1/8 tsp Coconut Extract

Directions

1. Combine coconut milk, tofu, 1/2 cup raspberries, sugar substitute (if desired) and coconut extract in a blender; blend until smooth. (If you want to remove the seeds, you can strain the mixture through a sieve, then return it to the blender).
2. With the machine running, add 3 ice cubes, one at a time, and blend until smooth.
3. Pour into a tall glass, and garnish with whipped cream and raspberries, if desired. Serve immediately.

Nutritional Information

- Protein: 8g
- Fat: 27g
- Fiber: 4.3g
- Calories: 310

Truly Coconut Cake

Servings: 16 | Prep: 20 m | Style: American | Cook: 37 m

Ingredients

- 2 cups Unsalted Butter Stick
- 13 tbsps Xylitol
- 2 tsps Vanilla Extract
- 3 tsps Coconut Extract
- 6 large Eggs (Whole)
- 3 /4 cups Organic High Fiber Coconut Flour
- 1 tsp Baking Powder (Straight Phosphate, Double Acting)
- 1 tsp Salt
- 1 cup Coconut Milk Unsweetened
- 1 cup Dried Coconut
- 16 oz Cream Cheese

Directions

Xylitol is used in this recipe to decrease the net carbs. Please measure first 8 Tbsp and then 5 Tbsp; keeping them separate and then powder each in a blender and set aside in separate bowls. The granules tend to be large and don't dissolve as readily as regular sugar or other granular sugar substitutes. Sucralose may be substituted by decreasing each of the amounts used by about 1/4 cup (add 2g NC to the total net carb count per serving. Please note this will make it too high in NC for Phase 1.)

1. Preheat oven to 325°F. Prepare two 9-inch round pans with oil spray, cut out parchment paper to fit into the bottom of each pan, place the paper in the pan and spray it with oil. Set aside.
2. With an electric mixer beat 1 cup butter and then the 8 Tbsp of xylitol that was powdered until light and fluffy, about 3 minutes. Add the vanilla and 2 tsp coconut extract; blend to

combine. Add the eggs one at a time blending after each addition; the mixture may separate a bit at this point.

3. Sift together 3/4 cup coconut flour, baking powder and salt. Add to butter mixture and mix until thoroughly combined. Add in the coconut milk and 1/2 cup shredded coconut, blend until incorporated. Scoop into prepared pans and spread evenly with a spatula.

4. Bake for 35-40 minutes until cakes begin to pull away from the pans and are fully set in the center. Cool for 10 minutes in the pan, remove from pan and then cool on a rack. The cakes will be a little fragile so be careful handling them. Place cooled cakes in the refrigerator until ready to frost and serve. Frost just before serving.

5. Frosting: with an electric mixer blend the cream cheese and 1 cup butter until smooth. Add the 5 Tbsp of xylitol that was powdered and 1 teaspoon coconut extract; blend until light and fluffy. Use 1/3 of the frosting to frost between the layers and the remaining to frost the top and the sides of the cake.

6. Toast the remaining 1/2 cup shredded coconut in the oven at 350°F for 5 minutes until lightly browned. Sprinkle coconut on top of the cake and along sides if desired. Refrigerate any remaining cake for up to one week.

Nutritional Information

- Protein: 5.4g
- Fat: 38.8g
- Fiber: 23.8g
- Calories: 442

Vanilla Mousse with Rhubarb Sauce

Servings: 2 | Prep: 15 m | Style: American | Cook: 10 m

Ingredients

- 2 stalks Rhubarb
- 1/4 cup Tap Water
- 1 tbsp Sugar Free Strawberry Jam
- 1/2 cup Heavy Cream
- 4 oz Greek Yogurt - Plain (Container)
- 3 tsps Sucralose Based Sweetener (Sugar Substitute)

Directions

1. For the rhubarb sauce: In a small saucepan, combine the rhubarb, water and strawberry jam; bring to a simmer over medium heat. Reduce heat to medium-low; cover and simmer, stirring occasionally, until rhubarb is a sauce-like consistency, about 10 minutes. Set aside to cool.
2. For the vanilla mousse: In a mixing bowl, with an electric mixer on medium-high speed, beat together the cream, 4 oz yogurt, and sugar substitute to semi-firm peaks. Reserve 1/4 cup mousse for topping.
3. To assemble: Set out two martini glasses or wineglasses. Spoon 1/4 cup mousse in the bottom of each glass and spread evenly. Top each with 1 1/2 tablespoons rhubarb sauce. Divide the remaining mousse between the glasses, then top with the remaining rhubarb. Top with the reserved 1/4 cup mousse, dividing evenly.

Nutritional Information

- Protein: 5.4g
- Fat: 28g
- Fiber: 0.9g
- Calories: 301

Vanilla-Almond Butter Cookies

Servings: 24 | Prep: 10 m | Style: American | Cook: 10 m

Ingredients

- 1/2 cup Blanched & Slivered Almonds
- 3/4 cup dry Whole Grain Soy Flour
- 3 tsps Baking Powder (Straight Phosphate, Double Acting)
- 3/4 cup Sucralose Based Sweetener (Sugar Substitute)
- 1 large Egg (Whole)
- 1 large Egg Yolk
- 2 tsps Vanilla Extract
- 1/4 cup Unsalted Butter Stick

Directions

This recipe is suitable for all phases except for the first two weeks of Induction due to the nuts.

1. Preheat oven to 375°F. In a food processor, finely grind the almonds with the soy flour, baking powder, and sugar substitute.
2. In a separate bowl, with an electric mixer on medium, beat whole egg and egg yolk, vanilla and butter until well incorporated (mixture will not attain a smooth consistency). With a rubber spatula, fold in soy mixture just until combined.
3. Form dough into 24 small balls; arrange on an ungreased baking sheet. Lightly flatten them with a fork to silver dollar size.
4. Bake 8 to 10 minutes, until set. Cool on baking sheets before transferring to a wire rack.

Nutritional Information

- Protein: 1.8g
- Fat: 3.9g
- Fiber: 0.5g
- Calories: 51

Vanilla-Bean Biscotti

Servings: 24 | Prep: 90 m | Style: Italian | Cook: 50 m

Ingredients

- 1/3 cup Unsalted Butter Stick
- 1/2 cup Sucralose Based Sweetener (Sugar Substitute)
- 2 tsps Vanilla Extract
- 2 large Eggs (Whole)
- 2 tbsps Sour Cream (Cultured)
- 3/4 cup dry Whole Grain Soy Flour
- 1 tsp Baking Powder (Straight Phosphate, Double Acting)

Directions

1. Preheat oven to 350°F. In a bowl with an electric mixer, cream butter with sugar substitute and vanilla seeds until light and fluffy, about 3 minutes.
2. Add eggs one at a time, mixing well between each addition. Scrape down sides of bowl with spatula.
3. Add sour cream and beat to combine. Scrape down sides of bowl again.
4. Add the soy flour, baking powder and beat on low speed until just combined. Chill dough for 1 hour.
5. On an ungreased baking sheet, form dough into a 12 by 2 inch log, shaping with moist fingertips if necessary. Bake log until almost firm, about 30-35 minutes. Transfer baking sheet to rack and cool for 10 minutes.
6. Using a serrated knife, carefully cut log crosswise into -inch-thick slices. Arrange slices, cut side down, on baking sheet. Bake at 325° for 17-20 minutes, until firm and crisp. Cool completely on baking sheet on wire rack.

Nutritional Information

- Protein: 1.5g

- Fat: 3.7g
- Fiber: 0.3g
- Calories: 45

Vanilla-Coconut Ice Cream

Servings: 8 | Prep: 240 m | Style: Italian | Cook: 5 m

Ingredients

- 1 cup Dried Coconut
- 6 large Egg Yolks
- 3/4 cup Sucralose Based Sweetener (Sugar Substitute)
- 2 cups Heavy Cream
- 1 14 oz can Coconut Cream
- 2 tsps Coconut Extract
- 1 tsp Vanilla Extract
- 1/4 tsp Salt

Directions

1. Toast coconut in an over at 350°F for 5-7 minutes - stirring halfway though. Remove from oven and set aside.
2. In a medium bowl, whisk yolks and sugar substitute to combine.
3. In a medium pot, bring heavy cream to a simmer over medium-high heat. Slowly pour one cup cream into yolk mixture, whisking constantly. Pour yolk mixture back into pot. This process is known as tempering.
4. Cook, stirring constantly over medium heat, until mixture is thick enough to coat the back of a spoon, approximantely 3-5 minutes. Remove from heat. Stir in coconut milk, coconut and vanilla extracts, and salt. Chill 4 hours.

5. Pour ice cream mix into ice cream maker. Process according to manufacturer's directions. About 5 minutes before ice cream is finished, add the toasted coconut.

Nutritional Information

- Protein: 4.9g
- Fat: 43.1g
- Fiber: 1.3g
- Calories: 435

Vegan Coconut-Vanilla Shake

Servings: 4 | Prep: 5 m | Style: American

Ingredients

- 1 14 oz can Coconut Cream
- 3 heaping scoops Soy Protein Powder
- 1/2 tsp Vanilla Extract

Directions

1. Combine coconut milk, soy protein powder, and extract in a blender and blend until smooth.

Nutritional Information

- Protein: 19.7g
- Fat: 21.2g
- Fiber: 0g
- Calories: 268

Walnut Blondies

Servings: 12 | Prep: 20 m | Style: American | Cook: 14 m

Ingredients

- 1 cup chopped English Walnuts
- 1 cup Unsalted Butter Stick
- 1 cup Sucralose Based Sweetener (Sugar Substitute)
- 1 tsp Vanilla Extract
- 1 cup Whole Grain Soy Flour
- 1/2 cup 100% Stone Ground Whole Wheat Pastry Flour
- 1 oz Vital Wheat Gluten
- 3 large Eggs (Whole)
- 1 1/2 tsps Baking Powder (Straight Phosphate, Double Acting)
- 1/2 tsp Cinnamon
- 1 square Unsweetened Baking Chocolate Squares

Directions

1. Heat oven to 325°F. Toast walnuts on a sheet pan for 8-10 minutes, cool and then coarsely chop. Set aside.
2. Line a 13-by-9-inch baking pan with aluminum foil extending 2 inches over both short sides of pan. Grease foil, and set aside.
3. Whisk butter, sugar substitute, eggs and vanilla extract together in a large bowl. In another bowl whisk flours, gluten, baking powder and cinnamon together; stir into butter mixture until well combined. Stir in walnuts. Spread evenly into prepared pan. Bake until puffed and set, and a toothpick inserted in center comes out clean (top will not be browned), 12 to 14 minutes.
4. Cool completely in pan on a wire rack. Drizzle chocolate in thin lines over entire surface of blondies. Let stand until set, about 1 hour. (The recipe can be prepared up to this point, covered with plastic wrap and stored at room temperature overnight.)

5. Firmly gripping the foil on both ends, lift blondies out of pan, and place on work surface. Cut into 12 pieces, and serve.

Nutritional Information

- Protein: 8.1g
- Fat: 25.6g
- Fiber: 2.5g
- Calories: 296

Walnut Brownies

Servings: 16 | Prep: 15 m | Style: American | Cook: 25 m

Ingredients

- 1/2 second spray Original No-Stick Cooking Spray
- 1 cup Unsalted Butter Stick
- 3 tbsps Sucralose Based Sweetener (Sugar Substitute)
- 4 large Eggs (Whole)
- 1/2 cup dry Whole Grain Soy Flour
- 1/2 cup Tap Water
- 4 oz Sugar Free Chocolate Chips
- 2 tsps Vanilla Extract
- 1 cup chopped English Walnuts

Directions

1. Preheat oven to 350°F. Line an 8 square baking pan with aluminum foil and spray with cooking spray.
2. Melt chocolate over a double boiler or in the microwave and set aside to cool.
3. With an electric mixer on medium, beat butter and sugar substitute until light and creamy, about 4 minutes. Turn speed down to low and beat in eggs, one at a time. Add melted chocolate and blend well. Add soy flour, water, sugar

substitute and extracts (3 Tbsp chocolate extract is optional); mix until just combined. Fold in nuts. Transfer batter to prepared pan.

4. Bake 20 to 25 minutes, until a tester inserted in the center comes out with just a few crumbs. Cool and cut into 16 squares.

Nutritional Information

- Protein: 3.9g
- Fat: 20.3g
- Fiber: 1.3g
- Calories: 217

Part 2

Introduction

You look at yourself in the mirror and through blurred vision, you perceive your body frame. You think about that lady in red and carelessly shrug your shoulders to your resigned fate.

Maybe your being overweight will never let you make an impression while your dumber but thinner counterparts get away so luckily. You need to do something about it and yet everyday when you lazily crawl out of bed nothing seems to right.

You don't want to go for a brisk walk or a jog around your block. You just want to creep under the rug and go back to sleep again. This way probably your day takes off. Then when you go off to office after hogging your unhealthy breakfast, you wish you had better exercised.

Somewhere in these entire daily marathon and other Olympic feats, you had felt that had you been fitter, life would have taken a completely different turn. Mornings would have seemed sprightly fresh, you could judge for yourself whether the clichéd statement-"Exercise makes me feel refreshed and rejuvenated" is true or not.

The office hours would have seemed better and better day-by-day, with people slowly succumbing to your popular nature. All these dreams could be true but first you need to create a good first impression. Lets us look at one the important aspects of this makeover program.

Nine out of ten times, it is noticed that an improper diet is responsible for the excessive weight gained by an individual. We forget the golden rule of "breakfast like a king, lunch like a queen and dinner like a beggar" and keep on piling the calories progressively throughout the day.

What we forget to pay heed to is that our body metabolism follows a certain pattern and if we go on disrupting it with our shifting eating habits, it will gradually fail and most of the calories ingested will get stored as fat in the body.

In order to redress the situation, Dr. Robert Atkins came with a miraculous low carbohydrate diet in the 1970's, which he elaborated in his book, Dr.Atkins' New Diet Revolution.

Although people didn't take to it then, with its re-introduction into public consciousness during the 1990's, it has become a matter of many coffee table discussions.

The Atkins diet has proved to be beneficial in many cases while nutritionists and health experts have exorcised it of all its fame and glory.

Chapter 1: background of the atkins diet

When Dr Atkins introduced the Atkins diet back in 1972, it created a worldwide sensation. Millions of people are ⬚uick to jump on the bandwagon and try this new diet for them, often with amazing results which further propelled the popularity of the new diet program.

Dr Atkins diet revolutionized the way people go on a diet. Instead of calculating the amount of food intake or calorie counting, the Dr Atkins diet works by limiting the amount of certain types of food while placing no restriction on permissible foods during the course of this diet of program.

Basically, this diet program is meant to be a lifetime solution and used as a dietary lifestyle that can give you lifelong weight loss solutions.

However, it is important that you get to know a few things about this diet program and discover the types of food permissible during the course of the Dr Atkins diet program.

The Dr Atkins diet program works by increasing the amount of protein rich food and limiting the intake of carbohydrate foods. By limiting the intake of carbohydrate and increasing the amount of protein, the body would be thrown into a state referred to as the ketosis.

This is the stage where rapid fat burning is done in order to compensate for the lack of energy sources when carbohydrate intake is kept a minimum level.

There are four basic principles that are responsible for the rapid weight loss and maintenance in the Dr Atkins diet program.

The first stage would be the most difficult to achieve but nevertheless it is the most important stage that determines the success or failure of your new weight loss program.

There are some views put forth by the critics of the weight loss program. Let's take a look at their points of view and decide if there is a basis for further considerations which may have been missed out by the proponents of the program.

1: Kidney Health

Some critics have been quick to point out that a diet that is high in protein would place considerable pressure on the kidneys to work twice as much as usual and this can lead to some undesirable effects in the long run. Possible damage to the overworked kidneys is one of the key points that the critics have raised during the debate concerning this diet program.

2: Unsuitable for Vegetarians

The Dr Atkins diet Is definitely unsuitable for vegetarians or vegan as it makes use of mostly animal based food to achieve the high protein count.

Even though there are some sources that comes from plants, but the major portion of the food included into this diet comes form animal sources, Therefore those who are vegetarians or vegan would not be able to follow this diet program.

3: High Fat

Diets that are fat-laden would definitely be rich in cholesterol and fats as well. Most critics argue that this is actually dangerous for the heart and for the blood vessel over the long run as excess fats in food and high cholesterol contribute to strokes and heart diseases while increasing the amount of plague in the blood vessels.

4: Low Fiber

As the Dr Atkins diet makes use of high protein food, there is a tendency to consume less food that is rich in fiber. This causes drastic levels of fiber intake that leads to constipation. It is vital to supplement the intake of fiber with supplements that would help replenish the lack of fiber in food intake.

5: Nutrition

A diet that tilts towards the intake of excess protein would definitely result in some form of nutritional deficit which is present in a wholesome, well balanced meal.

Therefore it is important to supplement this as well. The most common deficits found in the Dr Atkins diet is the lack of potassium and calcium which is essential for the normal workings of the body's metabolism process.

The history of The Atkins Diet goes back to the Dr. Atkins' theory that over-consumption of and hypersensitivity to carbohydrates is the root of our problem with being overweight.

The principle he based his plan on says that it is the way your body processes the carbohydrates you eat -- not how much fat you eat -- that causes you to gain weight. While most diet experts say that not everyone who has a weight problem is insulin resistant, Atkins says it is more likely than not.

By reducing one's intake of carbohydrates to less than 50 grams a day, one will enter a metabolic process called ketosis, which is nothing but a state in which one's body will start burning the fat to provide energy.

Atkins also says that ketosis will affect insulin production which will prevent more fat from being formed.

The Atkins Diet recommends exercise. Any diet that doesn't include exercise in its recommendations will probably not be as effective and does not encourage health lifestyle change.

Person suffering from gout, kidney conditions, type I diabetes or pregnant women should not follow Atkins.

According to some health experts, ketosis results in too-rapid, and unusual levels of weight loss and that the loss consists of lean body mass and water.

Regardless of whichever diet you persist on, be it be Atkins or Weight Watchers, diet experts agree that it is calorie reduction that results in weight loss.

After you lose weight, you can't just revert back to your original ways of eating crabs.

Remember, one should never start a diet without prior consultation to the doctor. This is pretty much essential with a diet like Atkins because it is so inflexible and is most likely a noteworthy change from your normal eating habits.

Additionally, some researches have indicated that this type of diet may endanger the kidneys, result in sunstroke, or lead to other health problems.

Before giving ATKINs a try, ask yourself: Are you committed to limiting your carbs for good? If not, then this plan probably isn't for you, because even as Atkins himself states, returning to your previous eating habits will bring the weight back.

Chapter 2: the atkins diet explained

Dr. Robert Atkins, best-selling author of 'Dr. Atkins New Diet Revolution', is the creator of the low carb diet craze that was re-introduced into the public consciousness 10 years ago.

His diet plan was originally created in the 70's and many people today have had great success in weight loss with his diet plan. 25 Million Americans are estimated to be on a low-carb diet at any one time. "Low-carb" products line the shelves of supermarkets as "low-fat" products once did in the 80's and 90's.

How does the Atkins diet work?

The first two weeks consist of a diet with only 20 grams of carbohydrates per day. This "introduction" period, as it is termed by Atkins, enables the dieter's diet to consist of meat, poultry eggs, cheese, butter, bacon, sausage, seafood and oils.

In these first two weeks, the dieter is restricted from milk, grains, breads, cereals, fruits or "high glycemic index" foods such as peas, corn, potatoes and carrots. In the next weeks of the program, the dieter adds 5 grams of carbohydrates to their intake per day.

In the 'maintenance' phase of the diet, participants are encouraged to stick between 40-90 grams of carbs permanently. This diet contradicts what major health organizations and health experts recommend.

The Atkins low carb diet, by nature, works by restricting carbohydrates. Because the body breaks down carbs much slower than other fuels, the Atkins low carb diet plan uses other methods of fuel that aren't in the form of carbs - so you can lose weight ⁇uickly and painlessly.

In simple terms, the Atkins low carb diet plan changes your body from one that uses carbohydrates as a main source of fuel to one that uses fats for fuel. Therefore, the body's natural storage of fat becomes the body's main energy source.

On the Atkins low carb diet plan, the body uses sugars as fuel. But, to turn sugars into fuel your body must use the naturally occurring hormone insulin. Insulin allows our cells to turn carbs into glucose (energy) by controlling the amount of sugar in our blood.

 Insulin causes the sugar we don't use as fuel to be stored as fat and it also keeps the body from burning stored fat. Because the insulin adds stored fats to our bodies, we're in a perpetual argument with our hormones when we're losing weight.

On the other hand, the Atkins low carb diet plan allows your body to release less insulin. According to Atkins, when your insulin levels are normal, you body begins to burn the stored fat as its fuel instead of looking for new fuels.

The resulting effect not only burns body fat, but it also leads to less hunger and fewer cravings. In short, the diet controls insulin levels by controlling the amount of carbs you intake.

The Atkins low carb diet plan consists of four phases of eating. The foods you eat depend on what phase you're in and your own metabolism. The phases include:

1. Introduction: This is the most restrictive phase, where you can only eat 20 grams of carbs daily. These carbs can only come in the form of non-starchy vegetables.

2. Ongoing Weight Loss: Phase two allows you to increase your carbs to 25 grams daily, and each week thereafter you can increase the number of carbs by five grams. You continue to add five grams of carbs to your diet until you no longer lose weight,

then you subtract five grams of carbs to allow you to maintain your weight.

3. Pre-Maintenance - This phase allows you to transition from weight loss to maintenance. You can add 10 grams of carbs weekly as long as you continue to keep the weight off.

4. Lifetime Maintenance: This phase allows you to select from a variety of foods while still maintaining a healthy amount of carbs. It's the least restrictive of all phases.

As you can see, the Atkins low carb diet plan is a rigid plan that many people use to great success. By limiting the amount of carbohydrates you intake in your system, you're allowing your body to use the stored fats in your body as energy.

This, therefore, promotes a healthy weight loss and if you maintain the diet through all four stages, you'll be healthy for years to come!

Chapter 3: advantages and disadvantages of atkins diet

No one would participate in any dieting plan without seeing the potential pros and cons of it. The Atkins diet is no exception to this and one should carefully research the Atkins diet pros and cons before proceeding with it.

Atkins diet pros include rapid weight loss, improved health, reduced risk of disease and methods to maintain weight.

But the most popular in the list of Atkins diet benefits is that of rapid initial weight loss, which mainly depends on a high-fat and high-protein diet that may lead to cons and may compromise a good cardiac and other organ health.

Atkins Diet Pros

Atkins diet pros are realized through the cutting down of the intake of bad carbohydrates into your body.

By significantly reducing the bad carbohydrates that you introduce into your body, it will start to burn the stored fat triggered by a processed named Ketosis. In fact, initially, practically all carbohydrates will be removed from the diet--not just those found in junk food.

You are basically consuming mostly fats and oils during the first phase. For most of us, eating high levels of fat is satisfying for us and causes us to lose weight faster. Don't just eat any type of fatty food however.

Limit the intake of trans-fats such as what is found in margarine and shortening. Stick to the good fats such as real butter, oils in nuts, canola oil, flax seed, and olive oil. Try to also stay away from the polyunsaturated fats other then those containing omega-3 fatty acids (like what is in fish).

Another of the Atkins diet benefits is the plan within its program to maintain the weight levels achieved. The idea behind weight maintenance is that each individual has a particular level of carbohydrate intake in which they will neither lose nor gain weight.

So after the initial phase of rapid weight loss, some carbohydrates are gradually introduced back into the body in order to determine what that level of balance is.

Another of the Atkins diet pros is the prevention of diseases such as Type 2 Diabetes. In simple terms, a high-protein and high-fat diet does not convert into sugar resulting in a stabilization of the blood sugar and insulin levels within the bloodstream.

Patients who are pre-diabetic can possibly avoid having to take insulin shots in the future by losing weight through the Atkins diet now.

One of the most pleasant Atkins diet benefits is the fact that you start to look better and feel better not only in your self-esteem but physically as well.

Patients who had chronic acid reflux and bloating from gas report that these symptoms begin to disappear once going on the Atkins diet. This is just because you are eating healthier and you weight is going down resulting in less pressure on your gastrointestinal system.

Atkins Diet Cons

The Atkins Diet is a popular and fast way to lose a lot of weight fast - there're many who give positive testimonials as to how much they did lose and how much better they feel. However one should be aware of the Atkins diet pros and cons before pursuing this diet.

This is why knowing the Atkins Diet pros and cons are so important! Of the Atkins diet cons, the often asked about is the danger of a high-fat and high-protein diet in relation to good cardiac and other organ health.

Affecting the proper functioning of kidneys is one of the Atkins diet cons not too often discussed. A measure of good kidney function is the level of creatinine in the bloodstream. A high creatinine level means that the kidneys are not functioning as well.

It has been determined that creatinine levels increase as a person is on the Atkins diet. Recommendations indicate that creatinine levels should be below 3.0. Any creatinine levels higher than that should be managed by a physician.

There is also the risk of calcium loss that is one of the Atkins diet cons. Calcium loss can result in the weakening of the bones or what is known as Osteoporosis. Osteoporosis is a loss of the healthy density in the bones and the bones become brittle and break easily.

If the protein intake remains high as in the Atkins diet, the calcium intake will be low. Reductions in bone loss can also be attributed to the ratio of animal to vegetable protein intake.

Another of the Atkins diet cons is the effect it has on persons suffering from gout. Gout is a form of arthritis and it is triggered by elevated levels of uric acid in the blood. The condition in the Atkins diet known as ketosis is where the body starts burning stored fat.

You want to go into ketosis or else the initial fast weight loss characteristic of the Atkins diet. As Ketones increase in your system, uric acid levels also increase and this is what complicates the gout.

Another common complaint from those on the Atkins diet is constipation. This is because there is a lack of fiber in this type of diet and fiber is what you need in order to give substance to a stool for passing.

You might need to take some fiber supplements to help prevent this condition. There is also the increase of the risk of heart disease because of higher cholesterol and saturated fat intake.

The Atkins Diet pros and cons should be carefully considered before determining if this is the right diet for you. It can be a very effective diet but just make sure it will not put you at unnecessary risk.

Chapter 4: the different phases of the atkins diet

It is too often the reality that millions of dieters the world over have won so many weight loss battles but always ended up losing the weight loss war. Winning the weight loss war is all about preparing, learning, and adjusting to overcome weight loss challenges.

This is to a large extent the way the Atkins Diet is structured through its different phases which allows for learning and adjusting during the weight loss process of using the program.

The Atkins Diet is structured into four different phases designed to help dieters achieve and maintain their weight loss goals.

1. The Induction Phase

This phase is obviously the most restrictive and eɗually most important phase of the Atkins Diet as it is designed to help the body break its "addiction" to carbohydrates. The consumption of carbohydrates at this stage is restricted to about 20 grams per day.

This initial restriction on the amount of carbohydrates that the dieter is initially allowed to consume is what most people view as constituting the Atkins Diet. This however is not the case as other phases of the diet gradually allow the dieter to increase the amount of carbohydrates consumed.

This phase has a list of acceptable foods with liberal amounts of protein including poultry, fish, meats and eggs, and also fats. However, anything that is not on the list of acceptable foods is strictly prohibited during the induction phase.

The induction phase normally lasts for about 2 weeks and as long as the dieter stays within the allowed carbohydrate food types and calorie limits, they are allowed to eat as much as they like.

This is however where caution need not be thrown to the wind because although the Atkins Diet is not a calorie-restricted diet, it pays in the long run to eat only healthy proteins and fats.

Weight loss during the induction phase is usually drastic due to a lot of physiological impacts of the diet. The weight loss experienced at this stage is however mostly body water loss due to the fact that the metabolism of glycogen for energy produces about 75% water which is subsequently passed out as waste in urine.

Dieters are therefore encouraged to drink a lot of water particularly during this stage and also during the other phases of the program in order to avoid dehydration and constipation.

2. Ongoing Weight Loss (OWL) Phase

The OWL phase of the diet is deliberately intended to slow weight loss in order to form the foundation for permanent weight loss management. This phase also gives dieters the opportunity to start tailoring the diet to fit their particular taste.

The OWL phase involves the gradual introduction of more nutrient dense carbohydrates into the diet. However, this gradual addition is advised to initially come from mostly vegetables such as cauliflower and asparagus, then from other fresh nutrient and fiber rich sources.

Also, the dieter is not allowed to add more than 5 grams of carbohydrate per week in order to determine what the Atkins Diet calls the dieter's "Critical Carbohydrate Level for Losing" (CCLL) - this being the daily threshold for carbohydrate consumption.

For as long as weight loss continues, the dieter is allowed to increase his or her carbohydrate intake by 5 grams per week until weight loss stalls, and then the dieter goes back to the previous carbohydrate consumption level.

The ongoing weight loss phase therefore allows dieters to eat a broader range of healthy foods including the ones they enjoy the most.

Also the diet places the responsibility of counting carbohydrate grams on the dieter and allows the dieter to discover what his or her actual carbohydrate threshold is.

Dieters using the Atkins Diet are encouraged to continue with the OWL phase until they have reached a stage where they are just about 5-10 pounds short of reaching their ideal healthy weight loss goal.

3. The Pre-Maintenance Phase

The third phase of the Atkins Diet is designed to help dieters prepare, acquaint themselves with and thereby have a foretaste of what the right eating habits of the lifetime maintenance of their ideal goal weight would be like. This phase is considered mandatory if permanent weight loss is to be achieved.

Once the dieter reaches the 5-10 pounds goal weight of the OWL phase, dieters would now be required in the pre-maintenance phase to increase their daily carbohydrate consumption by 10 grams per week for as long as they continue to lose weight. The idea is to continue increasing carbohydrate consumption until the dieter is losing less than a pound per week.

When a dieter reaches his or her goal, they are further encouraged to stay on the same level at which they reached their goal weight for another one month or so before increasing their daily carbohydrate intake by another 10 grams to see if they can continue at that level without any additional weight gain.

The dieter is to continue making the 10 grams weekly increase for as long as they continue to shed weight no matter how slow this may be happening.

The additional carbohydrate food helps to provide increased nutrition, variety, and culinary enjoyment making it easier for dieters to stick to the diet. This phase should last for at least a month but dieters are strongly encouraged to let it last for two or three months in order to achieve best results.

The goal of this phase is to help the dieter internalize the habits that are to become part of a permanent lifestyle as the dieter moves into the final phase.

4. The Lifetime Maintenance Phase

The last phase of the Atkins Diet known as the maintenance phase starts when the dieter has achieved his or her weight loss goal. At this stage, the dieter is allowed to maximize the amount of healthy carbohydrates he or she can consume from about 90 to 120 grams per day depending on the gender, age, and activity level.

The Atkins Diet is therefore all about preparation as it is structured around learning and adjusting to real-world challenges concerning effectively losing and maintaining healthy weight loss.

This 4-phase structure of the Atkins Diet is therefore deliberately intended to gradually help the dieter learn and also adjust his or herself to a new healthy lifestyle required to maintain the weight loss that the program has assisted him or her to achieve.

As the Atkins Diet rightly puts it "Maintaining weight loss is as much a mental challenge as a physical one." So it is important to keep yourself motivated while on the diet while also making sure to get adequate exercise.

Chapter 5: benefits of the atkins diet

You have a wide variety of diet choices, low fat, high protein, macrobiotic, vegetarian, the grapefruit diet, and the list goes on. So why should you choose the Atkins Diet? Here are 4 important advantages that put the Atkins Diet ahead of the pack.

Lose Weight Fast

If there is one thing more than any other that causes diets to end in failure, it must be going weeks at a time with very little to show for it. But not with the Atkins Diet. You will start to notice the weight loss in just a few days. Atkins dieters report losing 20, 30 lbs. or more during the 14 day induction phase.

Within a week others will start to comment on your weight loss. These results build your confidence ?uickly. You start to look and feel better. Your determination and resolve are at all time highs.

You will start to notice other health benefits almost immediately. Atkins dieters report shedding excess water, lowering blood pressure and cholesterol.

Easy To Maintain

The Atkins diet is, I believe, easy to maintain, maybe the easiest, since you do not need special meals, although low-carb options are available. Dieters generally have weaker and fewer cravings and are less hungry, because no foods are completely eliminated, just limited over time to a certain amount. This might even cause you to want to exercise more.

Burn Excess Fat Stores

An additional plus of the Atkins diet, and certainly the most desired by dieters, is this diet plan forces you to basically use your own fat to burn as energy. The process is called ketosis and it is the key to being successful with this diet.

This fat burning potential leads to obvious and fast fat reduction, giving you more resolve to see the plan through. A pleasing benefit of ketosis is that it also suppresses your appetite. This helps to decrease cravings and blast you to even faster weight loss.

Feel Full & Satisfied

Because of the wide variety of food permitted, you will feel full and satisfied. Once you get used to fewer carbohydrates, you tend to feel more energetic and less lethargic.

One of the delightful side effects of ketosis is suppressed appetite. Dietary fat also makes you feel full faster. You will say good-bye to cravings while enjoying delicious emotionally satisfying food.

When you choose the Atkins diet you will lose weight easily and faster than you can imagine. You will never have to fight off hunger. You will stay happy and satisfied, and the pounds will just melt away. The Atkins diet is your ideal choice for fast, long term weight loss.

Chapter 6: atkins diet food lists

Though the Atkins diet is not as popular as it once was, there are still plenty of people who are on it, and plenty more who still want to try to do it. There are some specific things you have to do to follow this diet, and you will need to know the Atkins diet food list before you can begin.

Unlike other diets, this one is extremely restrictive in the first phase, but broadens after just two weeks. Though it can be tough, there are many who claim it is very much worth a try.

When you first start, your Atkins diet food list will be very small. You will be restricted to some different types of meat, and a short list of vegetables. This induction phase has very little of any type of carbohydrates and is meant to kick your body into a different way of dealing with calories.

It should start your body thinking it needs to burn its food stores. You should start to feel better within a few days, and you might be surprised at how much you lose in the first week.

After the first two weeks, you will be able to slowly introduce some limited carbs. You are probably still avoiding bread and other processed and complex carbohydrates. By now your weight loss should slow down a bit, but this is how it is supposed to go.

Your body should be settled into a new way of processing your foods, and as long as you limit the carbs as you should be, you should be doing just fine. Many can't follow this because they love bread so much, and many other favorites are not included on the Atkins diet food list.

When you go on this diet, there are a few things that are more important than the Atkins diet food list, however. You have to remember that you should still keep your portions down to a decent size, and that you should cut out fats. There are some who go on this diet thinking they can eat whatever they want as long as they are not having carbohydrates, and that is just not true.

You should also talk to your doctor before you begin if you have ever had any type of heart or cholesterol problem in your past. Though this diet can be great to get your weight down, and to make you feel better, it can be hard on the heart if you have had problems.

The most important lesson to learn when it comes to your body is that it wants to have a boring and mundane existence. You may not believe me but if you have a pet, this is often one of the first fundamental lessons that the pet care guide highlights for their long-term health, are we really such a special species that this does not apply to us?

Keeping up with what you could and couldn't eat can be a challenge and that's why having an Atkins Diet Food List is necessary to help you stay on track. You simple look at which stage you are on and find the foods that you are encouraged to eat and those you are encouraged to avoid.

In fact, on the Atkins official site there are other free tools to help you keep track of your carbs and other food recommendations to help you to compile your own Atkins Diet Food List.

Helping You to Stay on Track

Protein

Protein is the main staple of the Atkins Diet Food List. You can eat all types of fish (salmon, sardines, tuna, trout, flounder and herring) fowl is also allowed (chicken, turkey, duck,) eggs, pork, lamb, veal, and beef.

Shellfish is also allowed but mussels and oysters should be eaten in moderation. Try to avoid processed meats like bacon and ham although they are on the list to eat in moderation.

Vegetables

You can eat several cups of vegetables a day. A good way to measure if you don't have a cup handy is to make each serving about the size of a baseball. The Atkins Diet Food List encourages a handful of vegetables over the others because they have a lower net carbs rate.

So that it doesn't get too confusing try to each all green leafy vegetables such as lettuces and cucumbers and stay away or eat in moderation the starchy kind, such as carrots, potatoes and yams.

Fruits

Good fruits to eat are avocados, tomatoes and olives. The sweeter fruits you can also eat in moderation except for the first phase.

Dairy

Yummy cheese is definitely OK. You can eat all types of cheese in moderation. However, ice cream and milk is off-limits.

The Atkins diet has shown how you can get great results with dieting and still eat tasty foods.

Chapter 7: steps to starting atkins diet

The Atkins diet is broken into 9 "rungs" of steps back to eating carbohydrates. The rungs are added in one week at a time during the "Ongoing Weight Loss" stage or "OWL" stage.

This stage is designed to allow each person to find their critical carbohydrate level for losing and to teach the dieter to eat these foods within reason, handle their glycemic levels and control cravings.

This phase begins when a person is within 10 pounds of their target weight. The rungs have to be reached in order but rungs can be skipped if you do not intend to include that food into your diet permanently, like the alcohol rung.

The overall goal is to add 5 net grams of carbs each week to your daily carbohydrate intake. Each rung incorporates 5 more net grams into your daily intake so by the end of the ladder you will have 45 additional net grams of carbs then you started with.

The first rung is adding more acceptable vegetables in higher ⬜uantities into your diet. This can be as simple as eating more salad or incorporating more cooked vegetables as side dishes to your regular Atkins meals. Keep in mind you are still limited to the introduction approved vegetables. The next rung is fresh cheese or fresh dairy.

Adding in more milk, yogurt and other dairy items to your diet while still following a more regimented plan. Some of the dairy options include hard cheese, cream, half an half, sour cream and low carb ice-cream yogurt and milk.

The third rung is nuts and seeds. Adding almonds, walnuts, sunflower seeds, etc into your meal brings in healthy fats and nutrients and are easy to incorporate into a low carb diet.

cooked vegetables or salads with nuts or eat them as an easy snack. You can find lots of great Atkins recipes for the new stages of your diet, with options to include dairy, seeds, nuts and more vegetables.

Berries are the 4th rung and include all types of berries like blackberries, strawberries and raspberries. Some limited quantities of melons are also allowed. AGR melons are allowed including watermelon, honeydew and cantaloupe.

The 5th rung is alcohol and includes low carbohydrate beer, white and red wine and spirits. Spirits do not have carbohydrate but low carb beer and wine do so choose wisely and keep portions limited.

Also it is important to remember that your body burns alcohol before fat so you can stall your weight loss by drinking too much, if you notice this refrain from drinking until you are back on track.

After alcohol you get to the legume rung. The 6th rung allows you to add in lots of different beans, humus and chickpeas, tofu and other soy products. It is important at this point you make note of eating higher AGR foods and make sure not to eat them alone because of their affect on your blood sugar.

Make sure to eat them with high fat and high fiber foods to minimize the affects on your blood sugar. Adding legumes into your diet is easy if you know the right Atkins diet recipes to follow, your new rungs allows you to incorporate a wider variety of tastes and flavors.

The 7th rung allows you to add in more fruits, in addition to the berries and melons from rung 4. Kiwi, apples, citrus fruits and

138

peaches are some of your fruit options. Continue to avoid dried fruit because they can be very sugar dense and in one small piece you may consume as many carbohydrate as an entire fruit.

Starchy vegetables are next and include carrots, squash and green peas. Corn and potatoes can be added as occasional treats. Remember to keep your starchy vegetables portions small. Finally the 9th rung of the ladder is the whole grains rung.

Make sure you keep your grains whole and unprocessed with small portions. You can eat oatmeal, wheat bran, low-carb breads and muffins, cooked barley and a few other whole grain options.

The rungs of the Atkins diet are designed to bring you make to a more normal eating plan, slowly reintroducing more common foods with higher carbohydrate counts.

It is important you continue to count your net carbs and keep them within your diet parameters to maintain your weight loss and keep you body at its new healthy weight.

Chapter 8: approved and unapproved atkins diet foods

While most diets center around what you're not supposed to eat, and there are some foods to avoid while on Atkins, this diet is more about eating certain amounts of specific foods at certain times.

The following foods are allowed at any time during the course of the diet, and may be eaten until you are satisfied. If you are someone who binge eats, and don't want to tempt fate with these healthy foods, this course on how to stop binge eating will get you on the path to sensible eating.

Meat: As long as the meat is unprocessed, it's OK to eat – beef, pork, lamb, veal, mutton, venison, and ham are all fine, as is bacon, as long as it's not processed with sugar (nitrate-free bacon is preferable).

Poultry: As with the red meat, poultry (chicken, turkey, goose, duck, pheasant, ⬚uail, ostrich, Cornish hen, etc.) is also fine to eat, as long as it is unprocessed.

Seafood: Like the previous two foods, seafood is OK as long as it, too, is unprocessed. Fish, such as tuna, salmon, catfish, trout, snapper, sole, sardines, herring, etc., along with shellfish, including oysters, clams, crab, shrimp, calamari, lobster, mussels, and scallops, are all fine to eat.

Make sure to stay away from processed imitation crab and other shellfish, as they contain sugar and additives. To learn which fish are best, as well as the most sustainable, this article on the best fish to eat will help you find edible treasures of the sea.

Eggs: All real eggs are fine on Atkins (chicken, duck, ▢uail, goose, etc.)

Next, we'll discuss some major food groups and how they fit into the Atkins diet.

Vegetables

Almost all vegetables, except for corn, potatoes, peas, and sweet and starchy veggies are allowed on Atkins. Vegetables may be broken down into two groups: salad vegetables, and other vegetables. Salad vegetables include:

• Lettuce (Iceberg, Romaine, Bibb, Escarole, Mache, Radicchio, Arugula, Endive)

• Leafy Herbs (Dill, Thyme, Oregano, Basil, Cilantro)

• Bok Choy

• Chives

• Cucumber

• Fennel

• Parsley

• Celery

• Hot And Sweet Peppers

• Radishes

• Daikon

• Sprouts

• Mushrooms

• Olives

• Jicama

Foods that fall into the category of "Other Vegetables", and are perfectly acceptable on the diet, include:

• Asparagus

• Cabbage

• Cauliflower

• Eggplant

• Kale

• Kohlrabi

• Tomatoes

• Onions

• Summer Squashes (Yellow, Pattypan, Zucchini)

• Okra

• Turnips

• Avocado

• Brussel Sprouts

• Leafy Greens (Mustard, Turnip, Beet, Collards)

• Broccoli

• Artichokes

• Fats

The best types of oils that you will want to cook with when on the Atkins diet are cold-pressed vegetable oils, and don't forget oils rich in omega-3 fatty acids.

Remember to stay away from margarine, though. If you're not quite up on the basics of how to cook when on a diet, this course on the fundamentals of healthy cooking will show you how to cook for a long and healthy life.

• Olive Oil

• Nut Oils

• Seed Oils

• Vegetable Oils (Cold-pressed)

• Linseed Oil

• Butter

• Fat Found On Meat

Condiments and Spices

Here is where you want to be especially aware of what you eat, as there are sugars present in many things people think are otherwise healthy.

As a result, most store-bought salad dressings are not Atkins-friendly, and your best bet is to make your own from scratch. This course on raw foods will show you how to make Atkins friendly foods, like dressings, sauces, and desserts.

• Salad Dressings – If making your own, keep it simple and healthy, combining olive oil with lemon juice, vinegar, or another tasty and healthy option.

• Spices – Individual spices are usually OK to eat, but be wary of spice blends, as they might contain sugar or maltodextrin.

• Condiments – Sugar-free versions of mayo, ketchup, and soy sauce are all fine on the diet.

• Sweeteners

Most artificial sweeteners are allowed on the Atkins diet, as well as one natural one (Stevia), but make sure to stay away from all natural sugars (sucrose, fructose, maltose, dextrose, glucose), as well as sugar alcohols (maltitol, sorbitol, xylitol), and honey and corn syrup.

• Splenda (sucralose)

• Stevia

• E?ual (aspartame)

• Sweet 'n' Low (acesulfame potassium)

Phase 1 – Induction

This is the strictest part of the diet, with only 20 grams on net carbs allowed per day. The idea behind this tough part of the diet is to ready the body to burn all the fat in the future Phases. You will also lose the most weight in this Phase, motivating you to stick with the diet on through to the end.

If you're one who eats when stressed out, and you're afraid this diet is going to send you over the edge, this course on how to stop stress eating will show you how to extract emotion from your eating habits.

In Phase 1, you must completely avoid all:

• Fruit

• Bread

• Grains

- Starchy Vegetables

- Dairy (Except Cheese And Butter)

- Alcohol

The Foods You Can Eat In Phase 1 Include:

- All Fish

- All Poultry

- All Shellfish (oysters and mussels are higher in carbs, so must be limited to 4 ounces a day)

- All Meat (see restrictions in previous section)

Eggs – Because eggs are a staple in the Atkins diet, and you may be eating them quite often, you may want to get creative when cooking them, so you don't get tired of them.

You can add veggies to them, or cook them in different styles, including deviling, frying, boiling, omelets, poaching, scrambling, etc, all of which are Atkins friendly.

Cheese – Cheese has about 1 gram of carbs per ounce, so 3-4 ounces of cheese a day is the max at this stage of the diet.

Vegetables – About 12-15 grams of your daily carbohydrate intake should be from vegetables.

beverages (club soda, caffeinated coffee or tea (1-2 cups), bouillon, no-calorie seltzer water, lemon or lime juice, caffeine free diet soda, herbal tea, water, bubbly or still (>8 oz. a day))

Phase 2 – Ongoing Weight Loss (OWL)

In the second Phase, you slowly start to add whole food carbs back to the diet, consuming a minimum of 12-15 Net Carbs daily, and increasing Net Carbs in 5 gram increments every week, two weeks, or month, whichever works best for you. T

Here is no set amount of time for Phase 2, and it lasts until you're about 10 pounds from your goal weight. The way the Phases work, is that you use the previous Phase's diet as a foundation, and keep adding to it, so everything in Phase 1 is still OK to eat.

• dairy (cottage cheese, heavy cream, mozzarella cheese, ricotta, plain and Greek yogurt)

• nuts and seeds (peanuts, almonds, cashews, hulled sunflower seeds, pecans, macadamias, pistachios, walnuts)

• fruits (blueberries, strawberries, honeydew melons, cantaloupe, raspberries)

• juices (lemon, lime, tomato)

Phase 3 – Pre Maintenance

Lasting roughly a month, Phase 3 allows for more carbs to be added to the diet, with 50-70 Net Carbs allowed daily. Now you're just 10 pounds away from your desired weight, and you are fine-tuning your diet, specifically your personal carb balance for when you are officially off of Atkins.

• starchy veggies (squash, carrots, baked potatoes, yams)

• legumes (black beans, chickpeas, kidney beans, lentils, lima beans, navy beans, pinto beans)

• fruit (apples, bananas, cherries, red grapefruit, red grapes, guava, kiwi, mango, peach, plum, watermelon)\grains (rolled and steel cut oatmeal, brown rice)

Phase 4 – Lifetime Maintenance

This is the fourth, and final, Phase of the Atkins diet, and should not be looked at as the last part of the Atkins diet, but rather the first part of your healthy new life. By this point, you should have your lifetime diet figured out.

You're at your ideal weight, and in order to stay there, a continued low-carb diet should be observed for the rest of your life, with around 75 Net Carbs being consumed daily, or whatever amount you have decided is best for you to maintain this weight.

In Phase 4, you don't necessarily add new foods to your diet, but rather, like we said before, fine tune and modify the amounts that you are already eating from the foods allowed in the previous three Phases.

All of the foods that have been mentioned thus far are up for grabs, and all that is required from here on out is the dedication to a healthy life that got you started on Atkins in the first place.

As effective as the Atkins diet seems to be, it allows for many different options when it comes to the foods you're allowed to eat. If your current, pre-Atkins diet includes a lot of breads and sugars, then you may have a tough time getting used to your post-Atkins lifestyle, but if you already have a pretty healthy diet, the transition to a low-carb diet shouldn't be too difficult on you.

And even if it is, it will have multitudes of benefits for your weight and your lifestyle, and going on Atkins shouldn't be thought of so much as a diet, but a lifestyle change.

Atkins recipes

Low Carb Asian Whole Fried Snapper

2 tablespoons lemon or lime juice

2 tablespoons sugar-free teriyaki sauce

2 tablespoons soy sauce

1 habanero pepper, diced

1 garlic clove, minced

1 green onion, diced

1 tablespoon diced lemongrass

2 cups peanut oil

1 whole snapper, gutted and scaled

Salt to taste

Whisk together the juice, teriyaki sauce, soy sauce, habanero pepper, garlic, green onions and lemongrass in a small glass bowl; set aside. Cut slits in the fish on both sides. Heat the oil in a wok to 350 degrees. Fry 6-10 minutes per side until crispy and golden brown. Serve with the sauce.

Makes 2 Servings

Carbs Per Serving: 5

Net Carbs Per Serving: 4

Low Carb Cilantro Lime Fish

6 firm white fish fillets

1/4 cup olive oil

1/4 cup fresh lime juice

1/4 cup chopped cilantro

Red pepper flakes to taste

Salt and pepper to taste

Place the fish in a shallow glass dish suitable for marinating. Whisk the remaining ingredients together and pour over the fish. Cover and refrigerate 1-2 hours, turning occasionally. Prepare your grill for medium-high heat. Grill 4-6 minutes per side to desired doneness.

Makes 6 Servings

Carbs Per Serving: 1

Net Carbs Per Serving: 1

Zero Carb Grilled Parmesan Encrusted Tilapia

1/2 cup olive oil

1 cup shredded zero carb parmesan cheese

Pinch garlic powder

Pinch onion powder

Pinch paprika

Salt and pepper to taste

4-6 tilapia fillets

Place the olive oil in a shallow dish. Combine the parmesan cheese, garlic powder, onion powder, paprika, salt and pepper in another shallow dish and mix well. Dip the fillets in the oil and press into the cheese mixture, coating both sides. Preheat your grill for medium-high heat. Place the fillets on a grill pan and grill 9-11 minutes per side to desired doneness.

Makes 4 Servings

Carbs Per Serving: 0

Net Carbs Per Serving: 0

Zero Carb Lobster Dip

2 pounds cooked lobster

6 bacon slices, cooked and crumbled

1/2 cup mayonnaise or to taste

Dash Worcestershire sauce

Dash Old Bay

Dollop horseradish

Salt and pepper to taste

Combine all ingredients in a glass mixing bowl and mix gently. Cover and refrigerate to chill.

Makes 12 Servings

Carbs Per Serving: 0

Net Carbs Per Serving: 0

Zero Carb Smoked Spanish Mackerel or Mullet

Simply tell your guy or gal at the fish market, you are smoking the fish so they can prepare it for you gutted and butterflied with the scales on!
2 Gallons Water

1 Cup Salt

6 Pounds Spanish Mackerel Or Mullet

Hickory Chips

Butter, Melted

In a very large dish with a lid, mix the water and salt together. Add the fish, cover, refrigerate and marinate overnight; turning occasionally. Soak the wood chips in water for 30 minutes and drain. Fire up your smoker to 225 to 250 degrees and add chips. Remove the fish from brine and pat dry. Place in your smoker scales side down. Keep your smoker temp at 225 to 250 degrees adding coals and chips as needed. Smoke for 4-6 hours until desired doneness (180 degrees internal temp) basting every hour with the butter.

Makes 4 Servings

Carbs Per Serving: 0

Net Carbs Per Serving: 0

Low Carb Ceviche

1 pound snapper, cut into small cubes

1/2 pound shrimp; peeled, de-veined and diced

1/2 pound scallops, diced

1/2 cup diced red onion

2 garlic cloves, minced

2 tablespoons olive oil

1/4 cup lime juice

Gently mix all ingredients in a glass bowl, cover and refrigerate overnight, stirring occasionally.

Makes 8 Servings

Carbs Per Serving: 2

Net Carbs Per Serving: 2

If you love ceviche, try all kinds of seafood combinations!

Low Carb Fried Clams

1/4 cup heavy cream

2 eggs, beaten

1 pound fresh clam meat

1 cup crushed pork cracklings

Salt and pepper to taste

Peanut oil for frying

Beat the cream and egg together in a shallow dish. Dip each clam in the mixture, then dredge in the cracklings. Season with the salt and pepper. In a pot, bring the peanut oil to medium-high heat. Fry in batches, cooking until golden brown.

Makes 4 Servings

Carbs Per Serving: Less than 1

Net Carbs Per Serving: Less Than 1

Low Carb Grouper Fingers

3/4 cup heavy cream

3/4 tablespoon distilled white vinegar

2 eggs

2 pounds grouper fillets

2 cups ground pork rinds

Pinch garlic powder

Pinch dill

Vegetable or peanut oil for frying

Combine the cream and vinegar in a small bowl, mix and let set for 10 minutes, then beat in the eggs. Cut the grouper into "fingers" and set aside. Combine the pork rinds, garlic and dill in a shallow dish suitable for dredging. Dredge the grouper pieces in the pork rinds, dip into the cream and dredge in the pork rinds again. Pour the oil in a fryer or large heavy pot and bring to 350 degrees. Fry in batches 4-6 minutes until golden brown, drain on paper towels. Serve with Low Carb Tartar Sauce!

Makes 8 Servings

Carbs Per Serving: Less Than 1

Net Carbs Per Serving: Less Than 1

Low Carb Lobster Salad

1 pound cooked lobster, chopped

1/2 cup mayonnaise or to taste

1 (7") celery rib, diced

1 teaspoons fresh lemon juice

Pinch Old Bay Seasoning

Pinch paprika

Pinch tarragon

Salt and pepper to taste

Combine all ingredients in a bowl and mix gently. Cover and refrigerate to chill

Makes 4 Servings

Carbs Per Serving: Less Than 1

Net Carbs Per Serving: Less Than 1

Zero Carb Parmesan Encrusted Tilapia

4 large tilapia fillets

Pinch garlic powder

Pinch paprika

Salt and pepper to taste

1 block butter, melted

1 pound shredded parmesan cheese

Preheat oven to 425 degrees. Season the fillets with the garlic, paprika, salt and pepper. Pour the melted butter in a glass baking dish. Sprinkle half of the cheese in the dish. Press the fillets into the cheese and turn over. Sprinkle the remaining cheese over the fish and bake 20-30 minutes until golden brown.

Makes 4 Servings

Carbs Per Serving: 0

Net Carbs Per Serving: 0

Zero Carb Balsamic Salmon

1 salmon filet

Dash garlic powder

Dash paprika

Salt and pepper to taste

1 tablespoon olive oil

1 tablespoon zero carb balsamic vinegar

Season the salmon. Heat the olive oil in a skillet on medium-high heat. Sauté the salmon in the oil until cooked to desired doneness. Transfer to a warm plate and garnish with the balsamic. Let sit for three minutes, then serve.

Makes 1 Serving

Carbs Per Serving: 0

Net Carbs Per Serving: 0

Zero Carb Blackened Fish

1 fish filet, your choice, at room temperature

1 teaspoon blackening seasoning

Salt and pepper to taste

1-2 tablespoons melted butter

Season the fish well with the blackening seasoning, salt and pepper. Heat a cast iron skillet to high heat. Dip the fillet in the butter, then cook the fish for 2-3 minutes on each side until blackened.

Makes 1 Serving

Carbs Per Serving: 0

Net Carbs Per Serving: 0

Low Carb Blackened Scallops

6 ounces scallops, at room temperature

1 teaspoon blackening seasoning or to taste

Salt and pepper to taste

1-2 tablespoons melted butter

Season the scallops well with the blackening seasoning, salt and pepper. Heat a cast iron skillet to high heat. Dip the scallops in the butter, then cook for 2-3 minutes on each side until blackened.

Makes 1 Serving

Carbs Per Serving: 4

Net Carbs Per Serving: 4

Low Carb Cajun Shrimp

1 teaspoon paprika

Pinch salt, pepper, onion powder, garlic powder, and cayenne pepper to taste

1 pound shrimp, peeled and deveined

1 tablespoon olive oil

Combine the seasonings and the shrimp in a large bowl. Mix and coat thoroughly. Heat the oil in a skillet and sauté the shrimp until well-cooked, about five minutes.

Makes 2 Servings

Carbs Per Serving: 1

Net Carbs Per Serving: 1

Low Carb Classic Tuna Salad

2 cups shredded tuna

2-3 hard-boiled eggs, diced

1/2 cup mayonnaise

1 tablespoon yellow mustard

1 teaspoon vinegar or hot sauce

1 tablespoon minced celery

Combine the tuna with the mayonnaise, then stir in the remaining ingredients. Serve wrapped in lettuce.

If you want, you can adjust the amounts of mayonnaise or mustard freely, as they're both CARB-FREE!

Makes 4 Servings

Carbs Per Serving: Less Than 1

Net Carbs Per Serving: Less Than 1

Zero Carb Crab Cakes

1 can of crab, drained

2 eggs, beaten

1/2 cup crushed pork rinds

Dash Old Bay Seasoning

Salt and pepper to taste

3 tablespoons peanut oil

Flake the crab, then combine the crab, eggs, pork rinds, Old Bay, salt, and pepper together. Shape the mixture into patties. Heat the oil, then fry each patty until golden-brown.

Makes 4 Servings

Carbs Per Serving: 0

Net Carbs Per Serving: 0

Zero Carb Dijon Salmon Bake

2 salmon filets

1 tablespoon olive oil

Salt and pepper to taste

2 tablespoons Dijon mustard

Season the salmon with the oil, salt, and pepper. Brush the mustard all over the filets, to taste. Bake in a baking sheet at 400 degrees for 14-17 minutes or to desired doneness. Garnish with lemon juice.

Makes 2 Servings

Carbs Per Serving: 0

Net Carbs Per Serving: 0

Zero Carb Drawn Butter

Serve this alongside seafood, particularly lobster or crab legs.

1/2 pound butter

Place butter in a saucepan and bring to a boil. Remove from heat and let sit. The solid milk will rise to the top. Skim it off and pour the remaining butter into a container.

Makes 6 Servings

Carbs Per Serving: 0

Net Carbs Per Serving: 0

Low Carb Fried Calamari

I don't know what people have against calamari. I guess squid is a weird thing to eat? It's perfectly tasty, though, and this preparation hides the squiddy look it has.

1 pound calamari, drained

2 eggs, beaten

1 cup pork cracklings, crushed

Salt and pepper to taste

Peanut oil for frying

Dip the calamari in the egg, then dredge in the cracklings. Season with the salt and pepper. In a pot, bring the peanut oil to medium-high heat. Fry in batches, cooking until golden brown.

Makes 4 Servings

Carbs Per Serving: 2

Net Carbs Per Serving: 2

Zero Carb Fried Fish

2 fish fillets

1 teaspoon Old Bay Seasoning or to taste

Salt and pepper to taste

1 egg, beaten

1 cup crushed pork rinds

Vegetable oil for frying

Season the fish fillets with the Old Bay, salt and pepper. Dip in the egg, then dredge in the cracklings. Heat the oil to medium-high heat, then fry until well done and golden-brown.

Makes 2 Servings

Carbs Per Serving: 0

Net Carbs Per Serving: 0

Low Carb Fried Oysters

15 ounces raw oysters, drained

2 eggs, beaten

1 cup pork cracklings, crushed

Salt and pepper to taste

Peanut oil for frying

Dip the oysters in the egg, then dredge in the cracklings. Season with the salt and pepper. In a pot, bring the peanut oil to medium-high heat. Fry the oysters in batches, cooking until golden brown.

Makes 4 Servings

Carbs Per Serving: 5

Net Carbs Per Serving: 5

Zero Carb Fried Shrimp

1 pound shrimp, peeled and de-veined

2 eggs, beaten

1 cup pork cracklings, crushed

Pinch garlic powder

Salt and pepper to taste

Peanut oil for frying

Dip the shrimp in the egg, then dredge in the cracklings. Season with the garlic, salt and pepper. In a pot, bring the peanut oil to medium-high heat. Fry the shrimp in batches, cooking until golden brown. Garnish with lemon juice and serve.

Make 2-4 Servings

Carbs Per Serving: 0

Net Carbs Per Serving: 0

Zero Carb Garlicky Blue Crabs

Catching blue crabs was always a fun outing for our family. I'm not sure if it was cost efficient, as we used chicken to catch the crabs, but it was certainly worth the money for how much fun we had. It's really easy, too. All you need is rope, a net, and chicken.

1 dozen blue crabs, cleaned

1 teaspoon Old Bay Seasoning

Pinch garlic powder

Fill a large stock pot with two inches of water. Season the water with garlic. Bring to a boil. Coat the crabs with the garlic, if desired. Place the crabs in the pot. Cover and cook for ten minutes. Remove from heat and serve with drawn butter.

Makes 4 Servings

Carbs Per Serving: 0

Net Carbs Per Serving: 0

Low Carb Grilled Parmesan Oysters

1 dozen medium oysters, shells cleaned and shucked

Melted butter

Zero carb shredded parmesan cheese as needed

1 teaspoon garlic powder

Place the oysters, still in the half-shell, on the grill. Mix the butter, parmesan and garlic together. Top the oysters with the mixture and grill for five minutes. Remove from the grill and serve.

Each Oyster Is 2.5 Carbs, 2.5 Net Carbs

Low Carb Grilled Salmon

1 salmon filet

1 tablespoon olive oil

1 teaspoon garlic powder

1 teaspoon dill

Salt and pepper to taste

Rub the salmon with the oil and seasonings. Place on grill at medium heat. Cook for 4 minutes on each side, or to desired doneness. Serve on a warm plate.

Makes 1 Serving

Carbs Per Serving: 1

Net Carbs Per Serving: 1

Zero Carb Shrimp Scampi

2 pounds shrimp, peeled and de-veined

Salt and pepper to taste

1 teaspoon Italian seasoning

2 tablespoons olive oil

1 tablespoon butter

Fresh parsley, chopped

Season the shrimp with the salt, pepper, and Italian seasoning. Heat the oil in a skillet, then add the shrimp. Cook until almost fully done, then add the butter. Add the parsley and serve.

Makes 6 Servings

Carbs Per Serving: 0

Net Carbs Per Serving: 0

Zero Carb Lobster On The Grill

2-pound lobster

Melted butter

Coat the lobster with the butter. Set them on a medium-high grill. Grill for 12 minutes or until red. Let set for 3 minutes and serve with drawn butter.

Makes 1 Serving

Carbs Per Serving: 0

Net Carbs Per Serving: 0

Low Carb Oyster Stew

For the oysters in this recipe, the ones that are canned or in the seafood section of the supermarket work fine. Just make sure you don't drain them.
12 ounces raw oysters

2 tablespoons butter

1 quart heavy cream

Salt and pepper to taste

Place all ingredients in a large pot. Cook over low heat until hot. Do not let boil. The oysters will be done when they curl at the edges.

Makes 7 Servings

Carbs Per Serving: 4

Net Carbs Per Serving: 4

Low Carb Oysters On The Half Shell

Raw oysters are kind of weird, in that they have carbohydrates, unlike most other raw animals. At 2.5 carbs per oyster, just watch how many you're eating

1 dozen medium raw oysters

Tabasco sauce to taste

Horseradish to taste

Lemon juice to taste

Using a shucking knife, open the oysters. Do this by sliding the blade into the oyster, then turning it sideways to pry it open. Place on a serving platter filled with ice. Serve with the Tabasco, horseradish, and lemon juice.

Each Oyster is 2.5 Carbs, 2.5 Net Carbs

Low Carb Oysters Rockefeller

To be honest, I'm not a particular fan of oysters rockers. I just find it so much easier to pry them open and eat them raw on the spot. That's not for everybody, though, so if you prefer them cooked and seasoned, this one's for you!
2 dozen medium oysters, shucked and in the shell

1 stick butter

1-2 garlic cloves, minced

1 bag baby spinach, chopped

Salt and pepper to taste

1/2 cup grated parmesan cheese

Arrange the oysters on a baking sheet. Melt the butter in a skillet over medium-high heat. Add the garlic and sauté for 1 minute. Add the spinach, salt and pepper and sauté until wilted, drain if necessary. Stir in the parmesan and spoon mixture over the oysters. Cook at 400 degrees for 20 minutes or to desired doneness. Remove from oven and serve.

Each Oyster is 3 Carbs, 3 Net Carbs

Zero Carb Salmon Cakes

1 can of salmon, drained

2 eggs, beaten

1/2 cup crushed pork rinds

Dash Old Bay Seasoning

Salt and pepper to taste

3 tablespoons peanut oil

Flake the salmon, then combine the salmon, eggs, pork rinds, Old Bay, salt, and pepper together. Shape the mixture into patties. Heat the oil, then fry each patty until golden-brown.

Makes 4 Servings

Carbs Per Serving: 0

Net Carbs Per Serving: 0

Low Carb Seared Scallops

Scallops are great! They don't really taste, feel, or cook like any other shellfish, which makes them uniquely tasty.
1-2 tablespoons olive oil or butter

2 garlic cloves, minced

15 ounces large scallops

Salt and pepper to taste

Fresh parsley for garnish

Heat the oil in a skillet on medium-high heat. Add the garlic and sauté for 1 minute. Season the scallops. Add the scallops, keeping them separate. Cook for 2 minutes on each side. Garnish with the parsley and serve.

Makes 2 Servings

arbs Per Serving: 6

Net Carbs Per Serving: 6

Low Carb Italian Shrimp Alfredo

1 stick butter

4 garlic cloves, minced

1 cup heavy cream

2 cups parmesan cheese

1 pound cooked shrimp

In a saucepan, melt the butter over medium-high heat. Add the garlic and sauté for 1 minute. Whisk in the cream and cook and whisk to thicken. Whisk in the parmesan until melted. Add the shrimp and cook until heated through. Serve over spaghetti squash or Zero & Low Carb Pasta and Rice!

Makes 5 Servings

Carbs Per Serving: 2

Net Carbs Per Serving: 2

Zero Carb Shrimp Cocktail

This is a dish all about presentation. If you've ever been to a really fancy restaurant, you'll know that presentation is 90% of a meal. This recipe is for one serving, so scale it up as needed.
6 shrimp, boiled, peeled, and de-veined

Carb-free cocktail sauce

Dollop horseradish

Chill a martini glass, spoon the cocktail sauce into the glass and add the horseradish. Arrange the shrimp along the rim of the glass. Garnish the center of the glass with a sprig of parsley.

Makes 1 Serving

Carbs Per Serving: 0

Net Carbs Per Serving: 0

Low Carb Smoked Fish Dip

I like this stuff too much. Whenever we got it as kids I had to be careful because I wouldn't even bother with crackers and just eat the stuff with a spoon. It really is a phenomenal little dish.

2 cups flaked smoked fish

2 tablespoons mayonnaise

1/4 cup sour cream

2 drops liquid smoke

1 teaspoon horseradish

Salt and pepper to taste

Mix all ingredients in a food processor until desired consistency is reached.

Makes 8 Servings

Carbs Per Serving: Less Than 1

Net Carbs Per Serving: Less Than 1

Low Carb Snow Crab Legs

Crab legs are a wonderful dish that's surprisingly easy to make at home. The best part is that it's eaten with butter, which is CARB-FREE!

2 tablespoons Old Bay seasoning

Salt to taste

4 pounds thawed snow crab legs

Clarified butter

Fill a large stockpot to half full with water. Add the seasoning and the salt. Boil. Add the crab legs and cook for 3-5 minutes. Serve with the butter.

Makes 2 Servings

Carbs Per Serving: Less Than 1

Net Carbs Per Serving: Less Than 1

Low Carb Steamed Clams

Everyone's got a different recipe for steamed clams. I prefer to make mine like you would crab, with the same seasonings. Try experimenting with different herbs and spices!
2 quarts water

2 tablespoons Old Bay seasoning

1 tablespoon olive oil

Salt and pepper to taste

5 dozen clams, washed and scrubbed

In a large stockpot, heat the water, oil, salt, pepper, and Old Bay until boiling. Add the clams and cover. Cook for 10 minutes. Discard any clams that haven't opened and serve.

Makes 4 Servings

Carbs Per Serving: 3

Net Carbs Per Serving: 3

I don't know why the ones that don't open are the bad ones. It's just common knowledge. Maybe they're just shy. Maybe it's so we don't have to bother opening them.

Zero Carb Steamed Lobster

Lobsters are actually kind of crazy. You put them into a pot of boiling water, then they scream and turn red and then you crack open their shells and eat them. It's brutal and delicious.
2 3-pound lobsters

Fill a large stockpot with salted water. Place a steaming rack inside the pot and bring to a boil. Add the lobsters on the rack and cover the pot. Let cook for 25-30 minutes. Serve with drawn butter.

Makes 2 Servings

Carbs Per Serving: 0

Net Carbs Per Serving: 0

Low Carb Tartar Sauce

1/2 cup mayonnaise

2 tablespoons diced pickles

1 tablespoon capers

1 tablespoon vinegar

Salt and pepper to taste

Combine all ingredients in a bowl. Mix well. Refrigerate and cover until served.

Makes 8 Servings

Cabs Per Serving: Less Than 1 Carb

Net Carbs Per Serving: Less Than 1 Carb

Zero Carb Tuna Steaks

1 tuna steak

Pinch garlic powder

Salt and pepper to taste

1 tablespoon butter

Season the tuna and let sit until room temperature. Melt the butter in a pan at medium-high heat. Cook to desired doneness.

Makes 1 Serving

Carbs Per Serving: 0

Net Carbs Per Serving:0

Low Carb Tuna Tartar

If you're familiar with Japanese food, you'll know that Tuna Tartar is very similar to a Japanese dish known as tataki. Make sure you get sushi-grade tuna for this dish.
1 pound tuna filet

1 teaspoon minced ginger

1-3 tablespoons soy sauce

1 tablespoon toasted sesame seeds

Trim away skin from the tuna. Cut it into small cubes and place into a bowl. Add the rest of the ingredients to the bowl and mix. Serve on chilled saucers.

Makes 4 Servings

Carbs Per Serving: Less Than 1

Net Carbs Per Serving: Less Than 1

Low Carb Land and Sea Salad

1/2 kiwi, thinly sliced

1 cup spinach leaves

1 avocado, halved lengthwise

1 grilled chicken breast, sliced

1/2 pound cooked shrimp

1/2 teaspoon black sesame seeds

Chill two salad plates, then arrange the kiwi slices around plates. Bunch the spinach leaves in the middle and arrange the avocado, chicken and shrimp on the plate. Sprinkle with the black sesame seeds and serve with your favorite low carb salad dressing.

Makes 2 Servings

Carbs Per Serving: 12

Net Carbs Per Serving: 4

Low Carb Australian Style Snapper

4 thick snapper fish fillets or other firm fish

2 tablespoon vegetable oil

Dash garlic & onion powder

Salt & pepper to taste

2 tablespoons butter

2 garlic cloves, minced

1 cup sliced mushrooms

1 cup parmesan cheese, shredded

4 cherry tomatoes, sliced

Fresh basil leaves and thyme for garnish

Preheat your oven to 450 degrees. Brush the snapper filets with the vegetable oil and season with the garlic powder, onion powder, salt and pepper. Arrange the fish in a glass baking dish. Melt the butter in a medium skillet over medium-high heat. Add the garlic and sauté for 1 minute. Add the mushrooms and sauté until tender. Spoon the mixture evenly over the fish, sprinkle with the cheese and arrange tomatoes on top. Bake 18-22 minutes until the fish flakes easily. Garnish with the basil and thyme when serving.

Makes 4 Servings

Carbs Per Serving: 6

Net Carbs Per Serving: 5

Low Carb French Baked Scallops

Olive oil

6 tablespoons butter, divided

2 pounds scallops

2 garlic cloves, minced

2 tablespoons green onions, chopped

1 ounce fresh lemon juice

Fresh parsley for garnish

Preheat oven to 375 degrees. Brush a glass casserole dish with the oil and arrange the scallops in the dish. Melt half of the butter in a heavy saucepan over medium-high heat. Add the garlic and onions and sauté until soft; pour evenly over scallops. Add the lemon juice and the remaining butter to the saucepan and whisk together until melted; pour over the scallops. Bake for about 15 minutes or until the scallops are done. Garnish with the parsley when serving.

Makes 6 Servings

Carbs Per Serving: 1

Net Carbs Per Serving: 1

Low Carb African Fried Fish Balls

1-2 pounds cooked fish fillets

1/2 cup chopped onions

2 garlic cloves, minced

Pinch African Berbere

Salt and pepper to taste

2 cups Zero Carb Pork Panko

Peanut oil for frying

Flake the cooked fish and place in a medium mixing bowl. Add the onions, garlic, Berbere, salt and pepper and mix gently. Add enough pork panko to thicken and place the remaining panko in a shallow dish. Form your mixture into balls and roll in the panko. Place on a platter and put in the freezer for 20 minutes. Heat the oil in a fryer or large pot and bring to 350 degrees. Add the fish balls and fry until golden brown. Drain on paper towels and serve hot.

Makes 12 Servings

Carbs Per Serving: 1

Net Carbs Per Serving: 1

Conclusion

When a person cuts back on carbohydrates in a severe way the body goes into what is called ketosis. Ketosis is when the body starts to use the stored fat for energy. This leads to eating less because you feel less hungry but it also has side effects such as constipation and not so nice smelling breath.

So instead of eating all the high filled carbohydrate food to get energy you would eat food with very little carbohydrates and start burning up the fat you intake for energy instead of the fat finding it's place in your body to stay like the thighs, butt, and stomach.

People who undertake the Dr. Atkins Diet plan are allowed up to 40 grams of carbohydrates per day. Since they won't be getting them from vegetables and fruit it is suggested to take vitamins to supplement what you would otherwise get from eating them.

This particular diet plan does not tend to worry too much about exercise being a part of the overhaul but it is suggested that some people may need to include this as part of their routine to get the ketosis state started.

The first two weeks of the Atkins diet plan restricts carbohydrates in the form of white flour, refined sugar, milk, or white rice. Basically the first two weeks are pretty much salads in some form.

After the two week induction phase you can then start to add foods back into the diet, such as fruits and vegetables, but white flour is absolutely not allowed at all for the length of the plan. As long as the weight loss is maintained then eventually you are allowed to increase the intake of carbohydrates.

The Atkins diet does work for losing weight and for better triglycerides and cholesterol but experts are very concerned with the overall safety of the diet, especially for those who have liver and kidney problems existing.

Like with any other diet make sure to consult your physician to make sure your body is able to handle the restrictions and have check ups to make sure that you are remaining healthy and do not have any negative health issues arise.